FROM
PSYCHE TO SOMA
AND BACK

FROM

PSYCHE TO SOMA

AND BACK

Tales of Biopsychosocial
Medicine

George Freeman Solomon, M.D.

with

Ping Ho, M.A.

1494-SOLO

Library of Congress Number: 00-191163
ISBN #:   Hardcover   0-7388-2325-2
                  Softcover   0-7388-2326-0

This book was printed in the United States of America.

To order additional copies of this book, contact:
Xlibris Corporation
1-888-7-XLIBRIS
www.Xlibris.com
Orders@Xlibris.com

CONTENTS

PART II

PSYCHOSOCIAL

To the late Joseph C. Solomon,
Ruth Freeman Solomon, and Paul C. Smith,
who have had the greatest influence on my development,
and to Susan Keran Solomon,
who is able to put up with me and love me.

INTRODUCTION

One must harbor chaos within oneself
to give birth to a dancing star.

Nietzsche

My mind kept wandering as I sat grieving in UCLA's Royce Hall on January 17, 1991, amidst tributes to my recently deceased friend and sponsor Norman Cousins, who had been a source of intellectual, moral, and professional support. The accolades of the speakers—deans, foundation presidents, and, most movingly, Shigeko Sasamori, the "Hiroshima maiden" Norman and Ellen had adopted—drifted in and out of my consciousness. Their accounts attested to the fact that Norman was perhaps the Renaissance man of our times: journalist, photographer, editor, advisor to presidents, behind-the-scenes negotiator with heads of state, intimate of the great and famous, healer of self and others, and challenger of modern medicine. Scenes from my own professional life intruded as I listened: . . . A lovely lady dying of lupus says to me, "If I had only worked with you sooner, perhaps it wouldn't have come to this." . . . An authority on immunology tells me, "Perhaps you should seek psychiatric consultation from a colleague. The immune system does not respond to emotions; it responds to antigens."

My mind continued to leap: . . . A young Marine sobs as he tells of fragging his sergeant after, on the sergeant's orders, killing a 14-year-old Vietnamese virgin who had refused sex with the sergeant . . . "How can I live with myself, knowing what I have done?" . . . A wave of nausea hits me as I recall the vivid description of necrophilia and dismemberment during my "truth serum" interview of a serial killer . . .

I had better get control of my thoughts! What would I say about Norman if called upon? I would say that Norman's "patient" was the ailing medical profession itself. What would be his prescription? First: to teach patients to become actively involved in their medical treatment process and to cease putting up with being treated as cases to be bled, probed, scoped, and scanned. Second: to humanize medical education. Third: to prove that attitudes and feelings influence healing and recovery through the field of psychoneuroimmunology (PNI), the field that aims to unravel the underlying biological mechanisms linking brain and body and the area in which I had invested so much of my professional life.

Being a psychiatrist, I couldn't help introspecting about my wild chain of associations at Norman's memorial service. I, too, had been all over the professional map. I shared Norman's humanistic ideals and wanted to make the world a better place in which to live, while never losing sight of the need to help individual human beings. I, too, saw science as a means to serve human ends. A great many scientists I have known have been concerned about humanity, but haven't given a damn about human beings. I, too, knew the power of the "mind" to heal, the inextricable intertwining of mental and physical well-being. Norman had written 27 books ranging in topic from the pathology of power to the biology of hope. Perhaps I, too, should write a book. After all, my professional and personal life had been varied, interesting, and certainly controversial.

My first psychosomatic research began in medical school, luckily on rheumatoid arthritis, an autoimmune disease. Later, I collaborated with colleagues at the University of California, San Francisco (UCSF), and at Stanford to study the psychological factors in the onset and course of rheumatoid arthritis and other autoimmune diseases. I became convinced that the brain influenced or regulated immunity— the body's defense against infectious diseases and, often, cancer. But the dogma of medicine held that the immune system was autonomous and self-regulating. I noted a small abstract in an obscure journal telling how a Russian scientist, Helen Korneva, had placed small lesions in a tiny portion of rabbits' brains that knocked out immunity. Little did I know that I would eventually engage in a collaboration with her and other Russian scientists that would continue for over 20 years!

Psychologist Rudy Moos and I wrote "Emotions, Immunity, and Disease: A Speculative Theoretical Integration" (1964). Very few believed us. If human observations were not convincing, I naively reasoned that animal experiments on the effects of stress and other experiential manipulations on immunity would be. Several years' work in what I called the "Psychoimmunology Laboratory" ensued, the results of which clearly supported our hypothesis. Science and medicine, however, remained intractably unconvinced.

Meanwhile, as Chief of Stanford's psychiatry service at the Palo Alto Veterans Administration Hospital, I dramatically came face to face with the psychiatric problems of Vietnam veterans, including heroin addiction. I wrote and spoke out on issues surrounding these problems in a number of forums, including national television, and managed to get myself on then President Nixon's "enemies list" (with interesting consequences which I shall explain later). Mardi Horowitz, a UCSF colleague now known for his research in psychotherapy, and I wrote a paper *predicting* the development of "delayed stress response syndromes" in Vietnam veterans. I helped set up the first treatment programs for addicted veterans, after initially bootlegging one against then existing Veterans Administration policies. All the while, I felt it important to be directly involved in the treatment of interesting patients, particularly psychotherapeutically.

In order to earn some extra money to supplement my meager academic salary, I took consulting jobs at the California Youth Authority and at a hospital for the criminally insane and for sex offenders. After the deaths of Martin Luther King and Robert Kennedy, a group of us at Stanford were prodded by some psychiatric residents to collaborate on a book summarizing current knowledge about violence. Its success led me to become an instant expert. *Then*, I really learned about violence. I was called as an expert witness in a number of fascinating cases, including several show trials, such as those of

Edmund Kemper, serial killer; Dan White, killer of San Francisco Mayor George Moscone and Supervisor Harvey Milk; and Leslie Van Houten, Manson family member. What could be done about the epidemic of crime and violence? Was criminality treatable? I *tried* to develop a model treatment program for criminal offenders. Although I refused to accept the impossibility of changing criminal thinking and behavior, I underestimated its difficulty. I became further discouraged by two attempts on my life (one foiled, as a knife was at my throat, by outwitting the hit man).

By this time, the field of psychoimmunology (now psychoneuroimmunology) began to take off, thanks largely to the conditioning experiments of my friend and colleague, Bob Ader. I wanted to return to the field, but no more rats and mice! So, what was the critical problem to tackle in 1983? AIDS, of course. I joined the UCSF Biopsychosocial AIDS Project, which helped to establish the relevance of psychosocial factors to the epidemic. After moving to the University of California, Los Angeles (UCLA), under Norman's aegis and feeling some degree of burnout in trying to figure out the psychobiologic aspects of what makes young people get sick and die, I thought it might be a research "upper" to try to figure out what keeps some very old people mentally and physically healthy. (Like AIDS patients, old people are especially susceptible to infections and cancer.) Might there be similarities between long-term survivors of AIDS and healthy elderly persons whose immune systems hadn't deteriorated?

I have, indeed, been a peripatetic psychiatrist. I believe that you will be interested in this scientific adventure story. This story, much like Norman's, is about overcoming resistance and indifference. My research has focused on finding linkages—usually unexpected—between one area and another, and pursuing those links.

I tend to take on what others haven't or won't. I have always had a facility for solving problems in novel ways, be they scientific mysteries or actual crimes. Obviously, these propensities relate to my own background. (How could I be a psychiatrist if I don't say that!)

I invite you to come along with me on this journey through medicine, psychiatry, psychology, immunology, war, and criminology. I hope you will find it interesting and fun. I did.

Although the journey may not seem like a physician's trip, it truly has been. In his brilliant 1960 paper, "A Unified Concept of Health and Disease," George Engel of the University of Rochester, both an internist and a psychiatrist, pointed out that *all* disease is *biopsychosocial* in nature. Narrow classifications, like "infections," for example, can limit complex multifactoral thinking. Rudy Moos, after parting professional company with me when I temporarily moved from working with people to rats, went on to do pioneering research on the *behavior-eliciting* (sometimes "sickening") nature of *environments*, including schools, hospitals, industries and prisons. Surely, the Manson "family" and the Vietnam war were powerful such elicitors!" If mind (brain) and body are inextricably intertwined, how could social influences on the psyche (behavior) be separated from those on the soma (body)? Unfortunately, inspite of its relative vogue, the *social* part has been given relatively short shrift by medical practicioners and researchers.

Perhaps you will find that there *is* an underlying theme to this book on varied topics, namely, the *vicissitudes of aggression.* Anger turned against the self, particularly when timidity or guilt have prevailed against standing up for oneself, may lead to an increased vulnerability to life crises-triggered, immune-related diseases such as cancer or autoimmune disease. In stark contrast, stored-up resentments taken out on others—without remorse—may preserve one's own physical health (at least when the death penalty is not involved!), but may cause suffering or possibly death in others. Being propelled by external forces to harm others *against* one's own inner conscience, however, may result in crippling posttraumatic stress disorder. The lesson I have come away with is: Don't let others screw you over, don't screw others over, and don't let others convince you that it is acceptable to do so when you know that it isn't. It may have taken a professional lifetime and research in apparently utterly disparate areas of investigation to come to these simple, obvious truths.

What next? It thrills me and gives me a feeling of pride to know that psychoneuroimmunology has exploded into a burgeoning field of investigation pursued by many able scientists; yet, I still feel compelled to do something unique and pioneering now that the field is in danger of becoming mainstream. When recently asked by a journalist, "What do you consider the implications of psychoneuroimmunology to be for the practice of medicine in the 21st century?" I replied, "Going back to the humane way doctors dealt with patients in the 19th century." Perhaps this book will help the reader to rethink the body and disease—even war, crime, and society. Whoever you may be, however, I surely hope that such approaches to come will be grounded in human values and based on evidence.

AUTHOR'S NOTE

Names and descriptive information about most patients are disguised to various degrees. Some forensic cases are undisguised, however, because information is in the public domain as a result of trial evidence. Colleagues are either accurately named, unnamed, or given fictitious names that are identified by quotation marks.

In keeping with the biopsychosocial model, the book has been divided into two parts: Part I **Biopsycho** (actually, tales of psycho*biological* medicine) and Part II **Psychosocial** (actually, tales of psycho*social* medicine).

CO-WRITER'S NOTE

Having singled out his name in a book nearly two decades ago, George Solomon was someone with whom I had always wanted to work. After receiving a copy of *Anatomy of an Illness* as a gift from my husband, Loren Bloch, I decided that the other person with whom I wanted to work was Norman Cousins. Tracing George from my own alma mater, Stanford University, to my own home base in Los Angeles, I called George, who referred me to Norman! The timing was right. Norman needed someone to serve as historian, and then Coordinator, for the budding Program in Psychoneuroimmunology at UCLA. In this role, I had both the privilege of working with George, one of the original members of Norman's Psychoneuroimmunology Task Force, and the privilege of being one of the last to work closely with Norman. (I collaborated in the writing of Norman's last two books, *The Pathology of Power* and *Head First: The Biology of Hope*.) By what feels like karmic fate, I now have the honor of co-writing George's book.

PART I

BIOPSYCHO

CHAPTER I

IN THE BEGINNING

The good practitioner must be able to bring elements of the body... into mutual affection and love and know how to create love and harmony among different elements of the body.

Eryximachus in Plato's *Symposium*

"Thank you, Mrs. Robertson, for agreeing to talk with me for a little while. I'm Dr. Solomon, a third-year resident in psychiatry. I'm part of the team here at the Arthritis Clinic, kind of unusual for a psychiatrist, but I have an interest in whether stress and psychological factors might play a role in some kinds of arthritis and related diseases. How do you feel about chatting awhile?"

"Okay, I'm glad to, Doctor, because I want to do anything I can to help figure out what's going on and because Dr. Engelman, such a fine man, asked if I wouldn't mind doing it. If he suggested it, it must be worthwhile; he's such a fine doctor, I feel honored that he's taken an interest."

"Well, Mrs. Robertson, I've asked to see all new patients who come in for the first time because of swollen, sore joints, that of course could be the result of several different types of problems. What brings you to the clinic?"

"Well, about three weeks ago my right wrist got sore, then swelled up. As you can feel, it's not only swollen, it's really warm and red. It is so sore I can't even write, and it interferes with my doing housework and taking care of my five-year-old. Now I'm *really* worried because my left knee started getting sore and stiff a few days ago."

"Has anything unusual been going on the past few months, any special stresses?"

"Oh yes, it's been a rough time. I separated from my husband a couple of months ago after a long, unsatisfactory marriage. Finances are difficult. I work part time as a nurses' aide in a convalescent hospital—I do really like to help people—but I have to take care of my son, and now it's so hard to make beds, serve meals, and so forth because of my wrist."

"Could you comment on the reasons for the separation?"

"Well, to be truthful, my husband is kind of mean. He'd never been warm or affectionate during our eight years of marriage. He has always been critical, jealous for no reasons whatsoever, and has even pushed me around at times. I got to thinking he was genetically incapable of love. I was patient and always hoped he'd learn how. But then he beat the boy just because he left his room a mess, and I won't let him harm the child."

"Could you tell me just a little about your own parents and early years?"

"Although I wasn't too close to Mother, she was a really good person. Very responsible. She put other people first; for example, she'd buy me and my sister new Easter outfits, even if she had to wear her own old one. My Dad was pretty strict but never mean. I was kind of a quiet, shy kid."

"Could you tell me the last time you got angry?"

"Actually, I don't get angry; my feelings get hurt."

"The last time?"

"Well, I must have been pretty annoyed when John slapped little Bobby around about four months ago."

"Can you tell me the last time you asked for a favor?"

"Yes, that was only a couple of weeks ago. I hate to ask for favors, but I did ask my sister to go grocery shopping for me. My wrist was hurting, and I was trying to work. She didn't mind at all, but I hated to burden her."

"Thank you very much, Mrs. Robertson. I hope that we figure out what's likely wrong with your joints soon and, after we get you under treatment, that prompt improvement ensues. If I can be of any help, if you'd like to talk further about those stresses, I'd be glad to see you again. It was very nice meeting you. Good Luck!" I encountered Dr. Epstein in the hall. "Oh, Wally. Could I speak to you a moment? You recently examined Mrs. Robertson. I just examined her. I'm guessing rheumatoid arthritis—not any other kind. Although I know that a definitive diagnosis can't be made yet, let me know what her x-rays and blood tests show. I bet she's got rheumatoid factor." [Rheumatoid factor is an autoantibody produced by the immune system that, like a soldier turned traitor, attacks a specific class of naturally present antibodies (immunoglobulin G or IgG), a common finding in rheumatoid arthritis.]

"I'll let you know. Somehow, you're managing to challenge my skepticism about all that psychological stuff. I have a couple of unusual cases you might like to see.

Mrs. Ethel Rosenbaum had married her college sweetheart, Mort, a good-looking, popular football player. But he never grew up. He was irresponsible, going from job to job with long gaps in between. He spent a lot of time at the gym, on the tennis courts, and on the golf course. He continually went out with "the boys", and Ethel wondered if it was always with just the guys. Ethel worked hard as a school teacher. Mort didn't seem concerned about her needs, didn't communicate. After nearly five years of what she considered to be an unfulfilling marriage, Ethel finally decided upon divorce. Before she got the courage to make the break, she found out she was pregnant. Ethel didn't want to be a single mother; she felt trapped. Rheumatoid arthritis ensued with an acute onset and in rather severe degree. A baby boy was born. Mort, who was present for the delivery, was thrilled to be a father. A marked change—belated maturation—ensued. He was a wonderful father, sharing care for the baby; he got a good-paying job in a financial institution and became involved in his work. Mort and Ethel drew closer together, really enjoying shared parenthood. Ethel's rheumatoid arthritis went into remission. Ethel proudly introduced me to Joshua, a friendly, lively, curly-headed four-year-old. At this routine follow-up visit, there was no evidence of joint inflammation; remission was complete.

Eileen O'Reilly, a pioneer in the women's rights movement, was executive vice president of a major national firm. She loved her job, at which she excelled. Her specialty was troubleshooting branch offices that did not meet national standards, a challenging task that would usually take several months to accomplish. She enjoyed traveling to various cities all over the country and in Canada. She made new friends easily, but never liked to get too close to any one person. A 38-year-old spinster, she attended mass two or three times a week and found the Church a great comfort. Her hobby was ballroom dancing, and she was good at it. Fortunately, every city had an Arthur Murray Studio, where she could dance and enjoy socializing. Tragically, it was in Atlanta that Eileen met a con artist dance instructor, a very handsome Latino of 35. What a charmer! Even though Eileen never thought of herself as pretty, Roberto fell head over heels for her. "Bobby" proposed marriage and pointed out that for only a couple of hundred thousand dollars (which she had in her savings), they could open a dance studio together in Mexico City. Although both felt that sex should wait until they were married, Eileen got pregnant. Roberto absconded with her life's savings. How could she continue to travel with a baby? The now desperate, pregnant "virgin" called her mother, whose response was, "How could you do this to me?" In the last trimester of her pregnancy, Eileen developed severe polymyositis, an autoimmune attack on muscle tissue. Eileen valiantly tried to take care of the baby by herself. I really liked Eileen, a truly lovely, brave person. She died three months later.

Such *nice* people were getting sick with autoimmune diseases when stressed and deeply troubled. Could such factors influence the immune system? How? I felt there must be more to autoimmunity than abnormal genes alone.

I had entered Stanford Medical School at age 19 in order to become a psychiatrist. On my first visit home after a few weeks of med school, I rather pompously asked my psychoanalyst father some psychiatric question. He responded, "Have they changed the curriculum? Are you taking psychiatry in your first year? I thought you were taking anatomy, histology, and physiology." My reply was a sheepish, "Yes, I am." He said, "Then be a good medical doctor before trying to be a good psychiatrist."

Fortunately, I learned early about the dangers of prognostication. While a clinical clerk on medicine service, I examined a lively, 85-year-old lady admitted for pneumoccocal pneumonia that was responding very nicely to penicillin. An Easterner, she had fallen ill while visiting a friend in San Francisco. She reported neither significant prior illness on "Past History" nor any major complaints on "Review of Systems"; yet, on physical examination, I noted grossly enlarged lymph nodes in the neck, axillae, and groin, as well as an enlarged spleen and liver.

I said, "Er, Ma'am, has a doctor ever told you about enlarged lymph nodes or swollen internal organs?"

She replied, "Oh, I guess I'll just have to tell you. I have lymphoma. Twenty-five years ago, the doctors told me I had six months to live. I ignored them. I intend to ignore you. Just clear up the pneumonia because I want to get out of here and get on with having a fun vacation with my friend!"

My first patient was a less-than-four-pound premature infant with a congenital hernia. I was horrified when told to "scrub in" for the operation. I had never even been in an operating room (OR). (I still don't understand why surgery was required so soon.) The surgical professor was infamous for ferocity and known to loathe his surgical assistant: a senior resident by the name of Conway who had been my feared instructor in dog surgery. The anesthesiologist had been unable to intubate the tiny infant and was using the ancient technique of open-drop ether—with problems. I was told, "Place your [scrubbed and gloved] hands in a sterile towel, shut up, and watch." I was most grateful to be relegated to the role of passive observer. The surgeon asked Conway, "I think it's a 'sliding hernia' [very rare as a congenital hernia]. What do you think?"

"I don't know."

"Why the fuck don't you look!"

"Because *you're* the chief, and if you don't know, how the hell do you expect *me* to know?"

The Chief picked up a handful of sterile instruments, hurled them in Conway's face and said, "Conway, you son-of-a-bitch, that's the final straw. You're fired! Get your fucking ass out of the OR!" Conway left (never to return to his Stanford residency).

The only scrub nurse present said, "Doctor, I've warned you over and over: I'll not tolerate listening to such profanity in the operating theater. I'm leaving!" She exits the OR!

I'm alone (except for the anesthesiologist) with the maniac surgeon. Abject terror sets in. My knees are shaking so hard that I can hear them bumping together as the Professor says, "Solomon, you will replace Dr. Conway." An early lesson in the sometimes-adaptive nature of acute stress response ensued. In spite of the premie's tissues tearing like wet toilet paper and my hardly being able to see what was going on in the little incision, I clamped; I tied. Sewing up, the Professor said, "Solomon, you're doing 10 times better than Conway!"

I decided to spend the summer between my junior and senior years studying medicine in England. I had the privilege of working with Professor John McMichael, co-developer (with Cournand) of cardiac catheterization, at Post-Graduate Medical School of London, Hammersmith. It was in London that I learned what really good clinical medicine and physical diagnosis were like. Unlike American professors, who tend to be called in only on the most puzzling cases and who see patients *after* work-up by medical students, interns, and residents, Professor McMichael took us along on his weekly clinic visits where he saw *routine* cases from scratch. "And what did your grandparents die from, sir?" asked the Professor. "Your pulse seems a bit rapid. Is there anything making you anxious currently? . . . Doctors, put your stethoscopes here where I have mine placed. Do you hear the slight accentuation of the second sound?" Professor McMichael didn't just rely on phonocardiograms and electrocardiograms (EKGs)—he listened to the heart and to the person.

We also had the privilege of being exposed to some all-time

greats: cardiologist Paul Wood, gastroenterologist Avery Jones, cardiac surgeon Sir Russel Brock, and hepatologist Sheila Sherlock.

It was clear that medicine had come to fascinate me. I was confused. Should I still go into psychiatry? Already, I sensed that there was a significant interface between the two. Of course, it was becoming more accepted that some diseases were psychosomatic in origin. The mother of psychosomatic medicine, Flanders Dunbar, by the 1940s had outlined personality profiles for people having a number of diseases such as hypertension, asthma, peptic ulcer. How could one make the psychophysiological leap from mind to body without abandoning the dualism between the two that had persisted since Descartes?

I decided in med school to try my hand at research. Moreover, I wanted the research to be at the interface of medicine and psychiatry. Research wasn't much encouraged in med school in those days, but one could devote a quarter of one's senior year for research. I asked my father if he had any research ideas. He said that he had had a number of patients with rheumatoid arthritis and was convinced that psychological factors were related to susceptibility and onset. (Little did he realize that he was planting the seed of psychoneuroimmunology!) "What factors?" I asked. He replied, "People may get sick when they stop being very active or athletic if they have used action as a mode of coping or defense by making pleasurable muscular activity." Dad had found that the onset of disease itself created a vicious cycle of greater immobilization and conflict that furthered the development of disease. I wound up doing a small research project on the topic, using skin disease patients as controls. I did, indeed, find that some very active people, like athletes or dancers, got arthritis when they quit the activity. They tended not to express feelings verbally but rather physically. The project won me a medical school research prize, which encouraged me to go on.

In those days (1955), a one-year internship (either rotating among specialties or "straight" in medicine, surgery, or pediatrics) was required before a three-year psychiatric residency. (I think it was a good system. I don't think the current four months in medicine in the first year of a four-year psychiatry residency is enough experience in general medicine for the future psychiatrist to understand the relevance of his or her field to medicine as a whole—which most don't.) I chose a straight internal medicine internship in light of the possibility that I would choose that specialty over psychiatry, and because I already considered it most relevant to psychiatry. My first choice placement was a prestigious East Coast program (Columbia-Presbyterian), where I thought my interview had gone well. The Dean at Stanford Med School had a different read on the situation, "You're not going to get it, George."

I asked, "Why not? I'm well into the top 10% of the class."

He replied, "First, Stanford—good as it is—is a West Coast school. Second, even though I presume you tried to hide it, they'll know you're interested in psychiatry. Third, you're Jewish. Do you want to stay at Stanford?"

"No, I think I should see a different—not necessarily better—approach to medicine."

"How about Washington University in St. Louis? They have a very strong Department of Medicine."

Thus, I wound up at Barnes Hospital for a superb medical experience that was an exercise in masochism. We were paid $10.00 a month—$9.95 after deductions. (Interns and residents make more now, but are usually saddled with big debts from medical school. They still work too many hours, although not as many as in the 1950s, to their own and their patients' detriment.) It cost $25 a month just to keep my car in the garage! We worked daily and every other night with one afternoon off every two weeks. Notwithstanding, the year (every day of which I counted in anticipation of its being over) left some incredible memories.

One day on rounds, we had the good fortune of having the visiting Professor of Medicine from Oxford as ward attending physician. A patient with a bizarre triad of symptoms was presented: peripheral neuropathy (impairing both motor and sensory function of nerves), myasthenia (weakness of the muscles), and a peculiar mental state verging on psychosis with anxiety, confusion, and paranoid ideas. The Professor said, "What did the chest films show?"

The resident replied, "They're normal."

"Let *me* see. Thank you. What is this shadow here?"

"It's a normal hilar lymph node."

"No, it's not. It is a small 'oat cell' (now called small cell) carcinoma of the lung. Only oat cell tumors produce that triad of symptoms. Take it out." The surgeons did. Symptoms disappeared. (We now know that such cancers produce a peptide, or small protein, called bombesin that is toxic to the nervous system.) Thus, substances made in different parts of the body, I learned, can affect brain and behavior—an important lesson for a future psychoneuroimmunologist. (I now like to lecture on "somatopsychic" diseases—physical conditions that can produce mental symptoms, often mimicking so-called "mental" illnesses.)

One of the oldest medical mysteries, which perhaps holds the key to explaining the role of expectations in healing, is the phenomenon of the placebo. In Outpatient Clinic, I learned the value of the placebo for the great number of patients whose complaints seemed to have no clear medical basis (and who, of course, never were appropriately referred for psychiatric evaluation). If the patient was tired or weak, I prescribed a (cheap) Nineteenth Century tonic: elixir of iron, quinine, and strychnine (a poisonous nervous system stimulant that was included in *minute* amounts). If the patient was "nervous" and had gastrointestinal complaints, I prescribed Elixir of Barhoma®, a mixture of a little phenobarbital sedative and belladonna, an antispasmodic plant alkaloid—cheaper than the essentially same Donnatol® and much cheaper and safer than the now vastly over-prescribed Valium® or Xanax®. (In those days, patients paid for their own medicine, and doctors were more aware of the cost of pharmaceuticals.)

When I was in Outpatient Clinic, the Social Service Department did an interesting project; they weighed all outpatient charts. For patients whose charts weighed over five pounds, they made a home visit. What they found, in general, were severely troubled, dysfunctional families. In those days—for better or worse—we could be rather coercive to patients, in part because Barnes was a private medical center. For example, an extremely obese person with hypertension, diabetes, and low back pain could be told, "If you don't lose five pounds by the time of your next visit in a month, your clinic card will be pulled." (In other words, "We can't help you if you don't help yourself.") A patient with emphysema might be told to quit smoking. What *wasn't* done was to provide psychological or medical support to help *enable* the patient to comply. Still, results were pretty good. Perhaps, some patients just switched to the not-as-good County Clinic.

Influential to my later thinking was a remarkable experience in somatic awareness that I still wish I could understand better. I now know that the immune system "talks" to the brain, but it still remains unclear how one can sometimes know what is going on in one's own body. I was at the weekly "CPC" (clinicopathological conference), in which an expert tries to make a diagnosis from the history, symptoms, and signs (like lab tests) of a patient who had died. Then the pathologist gives the real answer. That day, I noted that the psychiatrist wife of the Chairman of the Department of Psychiatry, whom we called "Mrs. Dr. G.", was there. Why was a psychiatrist at a medical CPC? The patient had been a Board certified surgeon practicing in a small city in Kentucky. He had presented himself at the great tertiary care medical center in St. Louis saying, "I have a carcinoma of the colon. I've come to your superb Department of Surgery, where I once trained, for a colectomy."

"What are your symptoms, such as bleeding or change in bowel habits, and have any tests been done?"

"I have no symptoms. There have been no x-rays, no colonoscopy, and there is no occult (minute amounts of) blood. I just know I have it. Do the tests here." Barium and air contrast enema x-rays were reported as negative; no bleeding was found; colonoscopy and other tests were negative. The surgeon-patient said, "Well, just take my entire colon out, do an ileostomy (that is, create an opening in the abdominal wall and bring the small bowel to surface to empty into a bag), and the pathologist will find it in the specimen." He was referred to Mrs. Dr. G., who had been told that the patient *definitely* did not have cancer of the colon. Mrs. Dr. G diagnosed a "fixed somatic delusion". (Delusional disorder is when a patient holds on to a false idea in the absence of other forms of psychotic thinking, as occur in schizophrenia.) For treatment, she recommended a unilateral prefrontal lobotomy! (I guess the surgeon-patient *must* have been crazy because he consented.) After his lobotomy, he asked, "*Now,* will you please take out my colon?" A second lobotomy was performed on the other side of the brain. The CPC, of course, was about the surgeon's death from metastatic carcinoma of the colon. The initial lesion was in the ascending (left) limb of the colon (which is an inverted U shape), a very rare site of a primary carcinoma and beyond the reach of colonoscopy. In retrospect, the radiologist saw the small (probably curable) lesion in the *original* films. It had been missed, and Mrs. Dr. G. had been misinformed. How the hell did the patient know? Indeed, there are a lot of hypochondriacs, but that case made me listen carefully to patients' opinions of their own illnesses.

As a final story from internship, I shall describe a case clearly illustrating the inseparability of physical from psychological causes of mental and behavioral symptoms. Fortunately, I began to question mind-body dualism early in my medical career, helped by having seen cases like this one. At Bliss Psychopathic, a distraught Mr. Jones brought in his wife for diagnosis and treatment. He had found her trying to light the bed afire, on which their three children were taking a nap. She had been a good, attentive, kind, never-abusive mother. There seemed to be no major problems in the marriage. Mr. Jones reported that the police had been looking for a firebug in their neighborhood because there had been several apparently incendiary fires (a fact confirmed by the St. Louis Fire Department). Mrs. Jones had no recall of any fire-related incidents and vigorously denied the possibility of trying to do anything to harm the children she loved so much.

Luckily, at that time, Bliss did electroencephalograms (EEGs) as a routine on-admission procedure in psychiatry. Mrs. Jones seemed to have a "spike focus" (abnormal electrical discharge) in the temporal lobe (a part of the primitive limbic cortex involved in emotions); yet, neither she nor her husband reported any history of seizures (convulsions, epilepsy). "Photic driving" was done to accentuate the mild EEG abnormality. The procedure consists of putting the person in front of a frosted glass screen behind which a bright stroboscopic light flickers, initially at 10 times per second—the frequency of the brain's alpha rhythm (that occurs in a relaxed, awake state)—and then gradually faster and faster. As Mrs. Jones stared at the screen while the bright light flashed faster, she screamed, "No! No! Fire, fire! Flames!" She then lapsed into a grand mal seizure (major convulsion). In her post-ictal (after seizure) confusion, she cried, "I'm sorry, Mommy! I'm sorry! I didn't mean to do it!" It seems that when she was five, while playing with matches, she accidentally lit the bed afire in which her baby brother was sleeping. He perished. The story was confirmed by her mother. The mother also reported that some time later in childhood the patient had an illness associated with a high fever, during which she had a convulsion—her only prior one.

Neurosurgery was performed. A small scar, which could have been caused by an old infection (encephalitis), was found in an anterior temporal lobe and removed. She was cured, and no further seizures occurred or fires were set. Evidently, during the seizures of psychomotor epilepsy caused by a focal brain lesion, the patient was reenacting a specific childhood trauma. Organic? Psychodynamic? Both.

I'd like to close the report of internship vignettes that had an impact on my subsequent professional mindset with a sad, humanistic story of a doctor's dilemma, still relevant in this age of high-tech medicine. My new patient at Barnes Medical Clinic was a very thin, gaunt woman in her 30s. Her "Chief Complaint" was, "I'm very tired, have been losing weight for months, and have hard lumps all over my body." Indeed, she had hard, enlarged lymph nodes in various sites and some hard lumps in the skin. Her rock-hard, knotty, and lumpy liver was enlarged almost into her pelvis. There were also palpable lumps in her abdomen.

I exclaimed, "Why didn't you come in sooner?"

She said, "My husband died last spring. I have three young children. We live on a little farm in Southern Missouri. I had to get the crop in alone so there'd be food for the winter." I was very obviously shaken. The patient said, "I've got advanced cancer, don't I, Doctor? I don't have long to live, do I? You've got to tell me because, if so, I must get back and find a home for my three children before I die."

I quickly said, "Please excuse me." I rushed out into the hall and then into the men's room, where I cried. Should I admit her for a biopsy to find out what kind of cancer it was? What was the difference anyway? Should chemotherapy be tried? (It was much less efficacious in the mid-1950s, and her disease was very far advanced.) If she got a lot of doctoring and died in the hospital, what would happen to her children? If I called the resident, wouldn't he surely hospitalize her? Who would pay the bill? (There was no Medicaid in those days.) Was there any chance of medical benefit? I went back to the examining room. With tears still streaming down my face (I'm starting to cry as I write this), I said, "Yes, you have cancer spread throughout your body. Please find a good home for your children. You're a wonderful, brave woman, and I feel very fortunate to have met you."

"Thank you so much doctor. I'll do what I have to do. Good-bye."

Did I do right? I still don't know. Is it not an advantage to a researcher of life-threatening diseases to have had *clinical* exposure to such situations?

My residency in psychiatry was at the University of California, San Francisco, the Langley Porter Psychiatric Institute. I had wanted to train elsewhere than San Francisco and not where my father taught on the clinical faculty. I went to Langley Porter, however, because they were willing to hold a spot for me despite my uncertain military deferment status. It was a good residency.

One of the best parts about residency was seeing each of our inpatients three hours (rather, 150 minutes) a week and really getting to know them. The average adult inpatient stay was six months (or *years* for autistic children, whose stacked charts could be yards high). In today's society, it's the opposite extreme. Who talks to inpatients other than to make the "correct" DSM IV diagnosis and pick the "right" medication and dosage—therefore, quickly to suppress symptoms and keep turnover high? What would the insurance company say?

As the reader already must realize, I refuse to conceive of virtually any disease as *all* biological or *all* psychological. The '50s were the heyday of psychoanalysis. During my child psychiatry rotation, the Professor analyzed the Ward Chief. The Ward Chief analyzed her assistant staff. The assistants analyzed the residents. I loathed inpatient child psychiatry because of the Professor's evangelical preoccupation with understanding *the* psychodynamics of autism (Kanner's disease). He thought that it was entirely caused by cold, emotionally unresponsive parents. I think I'd get cold, too, if my little child screamed every time I went near or tried to pick it up! Autistic patients and their parents were treated purely psychotherapeutically for years and years, generally to no avail other than exacerbating parental guilt. One resident bragged to me that he had not discussed any child patient in his six months there. The supervisor was more absorbed with how the *resident* felt about the kid defecating on the floor (that is, his own "anal conflicts") than *why* the *kid* may have pooped on the carpet (as if the pooping was supposed to stop automatically if the doctor were comfortable with feces.)

Each clinical case I encountered seemed to solidify my belief in the mind-body connection. An attractive, tall, slim, 30-year-old woman suffered from schizophrenia, catatonic type. Her response to the only effective neuroleptic available, Thorazine® (chlorpromazine), had been modest at best. She would speak only a few words or phrases, eat, move about, and dress herself. My thrice weekly sessions with her were most difficult—at least for me. "Good morning, Miss Johnson."

"Good morning."

"And what have you been doing in occupational therapy?"

"Knitting."

"What are you knitting?"

"Sweater."

"Do you like to knit?" Silence. Blank stare. Forty-five more minutes of her silence. Week after week for a couple of months. My supervisor advised, "Be patient." At this point, I must interrupt the narrative with a necessary personal note: During internship, I had fallen in love with a beautiful Danish postdoctoral fellow in hematology, who had come to the United States to study. We became engaged. She returned to Denmark. Our wedding in Copenhagen was scheduled three weeks hence when I got the "Dear John" letter. I had not sensed the premonitory signs (selective avoidance, no doubt). I was determined that no one would know how terribly upset I was, least of all my patients. The morning after having read the letter, I picked up Margot Johnson on the Women's Ward to accompany her, as usual, to my office on the Men's Ward. We were hardly out the door of the Women's Ward, when Margot turned to me and said, "You're terribly depressed today, aren't you Doctor?" The first complete sentence she had ever said to me!

In shock, I managed to lead her to my office. I said, concerned about being too personally revealing, "That could be. How did you know?"

"I really don't know how. I guess I just notice little things." (I thought, my God, that's what they mean by "schizophrenic's insight" in the textbook!) Margot asked, "Do you like butterflies?"

I replied, "I don't know very much about them, but I think they're very pretty."

"I guess I never told you, but my hobby is butterflies. Do you know that the beautiful coloration is often protective?" Thus began a long, almost academic, lecture on butterflies. The hour was almost up as I sat quietly in stunned amazement. Suddenly, Margot's blank face ("flat affect") softened into a smile. "Gee, Doc, I sure wish I knew a good joke." She was trying to cheer me up! Nowadays, such a "purely organic" schizophrenic would just be given the latest "third generation" antipsychotic drug.

While doing psychiatric consultations on medical and surgical patients, I had an experience more suited for a clergyman. I was asked to see a woman in her 30's, mother of two, who had severe mitral stenosis (narrowing of a valve between two chambers of the heart) as a result of childhood rheumatic fever. (Rheumatic fever is an immune disease, now rare because of antibiotics, caused by an immune attack against parts of the heart that are molecularly similar to a particular strain of streptococcus. Thus, the immune system mounts a "mistaken" attack on the valve after strep throat.) She had been on the surgical service, awaiting valve replacement, when she suddenly developed an active rheumatic carditis (heart inflammation) and heart failure. Surgery had to be canceled, and she was taken to the medical floor. The request for consultation was because of depression. I entered the patient's room to find her in an oxygen tent with Cheyne-Stokes (predeath) type respiration. I rushed out to find a medical resident. "You don't need *me*; she's practically dead!"

"I know. It's awful, but there is just nothing more we can do." I went back.

The patient gasped, "I asked to see a psychiatrist. I'm dying."

I wasn't about to argue. As psychiatrically as possible, I said, "You must have some feelings about that."

Mrs. Sutherland went on. "When I was a little girl, we were very poor, but we lived in a nice neighborhood. My friend had silk panties, but I only had cotton panties. One day when I was over at her house, I stole a pair of her silk panties. I was five. I don't think a day of my life has gone by that I haven't felt guilty about being a thief. Do you think I'm a terrible person, Doctor?"

I was aghast. "Of course not! That was just childish mischief like any five-year-old's. I'm sure you must be a very good person."

"Thank you, Doctor. Now I can die in peace." Gasp. Head back. No breath. Eyes rolled up. No pulse. Dead.

I ran out and grabbed the resident. Dead. Somehow, the patient had waited to die until she confessed her "sin". The power of the mind over the body.

Another case history involving rheumatic fever is relevant, if not to psychoneuroimmunology, to the currently controversial issue of euthanasia. A nurse in her late 20s named Elizabeth, formerly employed at the university hospital, was admitted for alcoholism and abuse of prescription drugs that had begun abruptly two years earlier. She could no longer work and was neglecting her small child. As Chief Resident, and her assigned physician, I wanted very much to help this attractive, bright, young woman whose marriage to a Chief Resident in another specialty was barely intact. I could figure out nothing. An only child of loving, older parents who had been thrilled by her birth after many years of frustrating childlessness, Elizabeth had perhaps been a bit spoiled. She had been popular, had done well in school, and had shown no prior psychopathology or signs of substance abuse. There was no family history of addictive illness.

Medical history revealed that she had suffered rheumatic fever as a child and had been confined to bed for a year. One day I said to Elizabeth, "Tell me about the *first* time you ever got drunk."

"It was the day Mary died."

"Who was Mary?" It turned out that Mary had been Elizabeth's closest friend. They had been roommates in nursing school. Mary had helped Elizabeth when her little boy was very sick and had been a companion while Elizabeth's husband was overseas on military duty. Still single and in her late 20s, Mary had developed a rapidly-spreading ovarian cancer. During the final stages, she had been hospitalized and had suffered greatly. Elizabeth had volunteered to be her special duty nurse, sleeping on a cot in the hospital room in order to be accessible 24 hours a day, having arranged appropriate child care when her husband was not available. Finally, Mary's agony became unbearable. There was no hope. Mary's doctor wrote an order for half a grain of morphine every half hour (a lethal dose), to be injected by Elizabeth.

As she told this tragic story, all of sudden Mary shouted, sobbing, "I killed her! I killed her! I was always jealous. She always got better grades. She was prettier. She had more boyfriends. She was more popular. I killed her, oh, I killed her!"

"But that certainly doesn't mean you wanted her to die. How did you actually treat her?"

"I tried so hard to help her, to be with her to the end."

I said, "In reality, I doubt anyone could have had a better friend." Elizabeth stopped trying to sneak drugs and began appreciating her husband and child. I knew that she needed more therapy for her guilt and related issues, so I referred her for outpatient treatment to one of my best former supervisors, a gifted woman psychoanalyst.

About a year later, my former teacher called me. "George, it saddens me to have to tell you that Elizabeth just died. She got a strep throat followed by a fulminant rheumatic carditis, and her heart failed." Would Elizabeth have died if Mary hadn't? I wondered. She had certainly been "heartbroken".

I decided to try a research project during residency to help me decide whether to enter academic medicine or private practice. I hooked up with one of my best resident friends, Bill Dickerson, who had become interested in psychiatry while a medical student at the University of Oklahoma. Together, we hunted for a project with both medical and psychological aspects. The search led us to UCSF endocrinologist Gene Eisenberg. Dr. Eisenberg was planning to compare the efficacy of estrogen (a female hormone) with an androgen-like drug (a synthetic male hormone with relatively few masculinizing effects) as a treatment for osteoporosis in elderly women. (Osteoporosis is the weakening of bone through loss of its calcium/protein matrix.) We would compare the psychological effects of both hormones with their physiological effects—a psychoendocrine project. We planned to use two controls, an inert placebo (sugar pill) and an active placebo (a stimulant-sedative combination then commonly used for mild anxious depression that would have no effect on bone).

We were very lucky. The pioneer in psychoendocrinology, David Hamburg, M.D., then at the National Institutes of Mental Health, was on sabbatical at the Center for Advanced Studies in Behavioral Sciences at Stanford. He had studied the relationship between psychological stress (such as having a terminally ill child) and the elevation of adrenocorticosteroid hormones. I probably never would have become a researcher without David's help. He was the perfect mentor for a young would-be researcher—affirming our creativity, guiding us constructively, never making us feel inadequate. Bill and I discovered that while estrogen led to both subjective and objective improvements in osteoporosis, the *perceived* reduction in discomfort was not related to the *actual* improvement in calcium uptake by bone. Androgen fortified bones, but produced malaise (and, in some old ladies, an unwanted production of sexual desire and dreams). Both placebos led to reported improvement in discomfort. In individual cases, personality was a greater predictor of perceived improvement than the nature of the medication. Our paper was published in a prestigious peer-reviewed journal—a triumph considering our mere resident status. I had found my niche in research.

Meanwhile, I had decided to put a different slant on my clinical work as well. Instead of doing psychiatric consultations on *disturbed* patients identified by other medical school departments, I decided to try to demonstrate the value of psychiatry in the care of *regular* medical or surgical patients. (This process is now more accepted and is called liaison psychiatry.) The Director of Residency Training, said, "Okay. What group do you want me to try to tie you up with? Cardiac intensive care? Medical oncology? Pediatric neurology?"

I replied, in what turned out to be a fateful decision, "How about the Rheumatic Disease Group? I did a research project on rheumatoid arthritis in med school." With some hesitation, the Rheumatic Disease Group agreed to let me tag along. For some time, the only patients they ever asked me about were those with major mental disturbances secondary to the severe autoimmune disease systemic lupus erythematosus (usually fatal in those days), in which the immune system produces antibodies and lymphocytes directed against components of the nuclei (DNA) of one's own cells.

Lupus-related psychosis was often mistaken for steroid-induced psychosis because lupus and other autoimmune diseases are treated by adrenocorticosteroid hormones which have anti-inflammatory and immune-suppressive effects. Corticosteroids are known to be able to cause psychosis. Yet, ironically, most of these patients' mental disturbances could be cleared up by marked *increases* in steroid dosage. Moreover, the very treatable and usually transient psychosis of systemic lupus erythematosus was often indistinguishable from schizophrenia—with both "primary" and "secondary" symptoms such as withdrawal, idiosyncratic thinking, disturbances of mood and emotions, ambivalence, jumbled thinking leading from one topic to another, delusions, and hallucinations. It occurred to me, "Could schizophrenia be an autoimmune disease of the brain?" I was already beginning to think psychobiologically and multifactorially. Just as autoimmune disease tends to run in families with a particular type of histocompatibility locus antigen (HLA), schizophrenia, too, probably has a genetic component. In addition, people with certain types of personality seemed to be more vulnerable to autoimmune diseases; the same seemed to be true for schizophrenia [witness the schizoid (loner) or schizotypal (oddball) types]. Furthermore, in many cases, stress seemed to precipitate the onset of both autoimmune diseases and schizophrenia.

Another reason to consider the role of autoantibodies in schizophrenia is their potential relationship to neurotransmitters [substances that carry signals across gaps between nerve endings (synapses)]. An autoantibody can act as a ligand, a substance that binds to a receptor site and causes its activation. Since schizophrenia appears to be related to an excess of the neurotransmitter dopamine, it has been suggested that an autoantibody in schizophrenia might be acting like dopamine.

Particularly odd in schizophrenia is the presence of rheumatoid factor (an antibody against an antibody, immunoglobulin G), that is found in most rheumatoid arthritics. About four times as many schizophrenics than normals have detectable amounts of rheumatoid factor—*but*, paradoxically, large scale surveys involving comprehensive examinations have shown that rheumatoid arthritis and schizophrenia do not appear to co-exist. *Other* types of mentally ill patients (affective, delusional, or demented psychotics) may have rheumatoid arthritis, however. Occasionally, a person who *had* been diagnosed with schizophrenia, but is not *currently* mentally ill, may develop rheumatoid arthritis, and a person with rheumatoid arthritis that is in remission may develop schizophrenia. Does this not all suggest that the brain and the immune system are somehow interrelated?

I decided to test the sera of some schizophrenic patients for antinuclear factor (ANF), the type of antibodies found in conjunction with lupus that targets cell nuclei. (Recall that lupus can be associated with psychotic symptoms.) I made a fortuitous mistake. (This one time, my meager "wet laboratory" skills worked to my advantage.) I found that 80% of schizophrenics had ANF! Because it took me a while to figure out that I had performed the test wrong, (about 5% of schizophrenics *actually* have this factor), I proceeded as normal. Among us, as a post residency fellow with the Rheumatic Disease Group, was the brilliant young English internist/immunologist, W. Jeffrey Fessel, the youngest person ever to have been elected to membership in the Royal College of Physicians. He and I had already published a paper on psychosis and systemic lupus erythematosus, reporting that mental manifestations could be the initial presenting symptom of the disease. "Jeff, would you consider coming to Langley Porter and working on autoimmunity and schizophrenia? We have a new research facility with an available wet lab. I think we can get some start-up research money. We might even start a new field, 'immunopsychiatry'!" With some arm-twisting, Jeffrey came to the Department of Psychiatry; however, my residency was about to end, and I was due to enter the Army. Perhaps, I could get an extension of my deferment. I got three months.

I was upset to be drafted just as the arthritis and schizophrenia work was moving along. Fortunately, in continuation of the work we had started together, Jeffrey and Japanese pathologist Motoe Hirata-Hibi identified anti-brain autoantibodies and structurally abnormal lymphocytes in the blood of some schizophrenics and their close relatives, work that continues and remains controversial to this day.

I was shipped off for six weeks of basic training at Ft. Sam Houston in San Antonio, Texas (1959). In those days, doctors had *real* basic. We marched, crawled under live gunfire, went through obstacle courses, and were left in the desert with only a map and compass. Goats were shot, and we had to debride (cut away) the dead tissue, the "war wounds". (I did not excel at goat surgery!) I thought it was stupid to use nail polish remover to strip the lacquer off a perfectly shiny brass belt buckle only to begin polishing it again. So I only polished the front. I got caught by the drill sergeant and had to march the platoon of doctors back and forth for an hour in the noonday Texas sun for punishment. I learned an important lesson. If you give the appearance of conformity, you can get away with a lot. If you're labeled a rebel, forget it. I became a spit and polish officer with shiny boots, a snappy salute, and tailored fatigues—attributes that were to serve me well in the military and, analogously, later in academic life. My truly rebellious, unconventional—even weird—nature would remain concealed. I learned to try to change systems from within—leaving the defiant approach as a very last resort.

I had no idea where I'd be stationed after basic. Naturally, I was hoping for Letterman Hospital in San Francisco's Presidio or Ft. Ord in Monterey. No such luck; it was to be Ft. McClellan in Anniston, Alabama. I had never heard of the town, located between Atlanta and Birmingham (which, in those times of horrible racial strife, we referred to as "Bombingham").

What proved to be the most weighty part of the military experience was my somewhat peripheral, but revealing, involvement in the Chemical Corps' "incapacitating agent" program. Somehow, after many months of investigation, I was given top secret security clearance. A funny story may account for this status. I was home from the Army on emergency leave to see my dying grandmother. While taking a walk near my parents' home, I was stopped by a man who asked, "Are you from this neighborhood?"

"I grew up here."

"Did you by any chance know a George Solomon?"

"I know him extremely well."

"Do you think he has any left wing tendencies?"

"No, he's rather conservative."

"Do you think he's a loyal American?"

"I've never met anyone more patriotic." (No wonder intelligence failed to foresee the fall of the Soviet empire!)

I had to sign a written pledge never to reveal secret information. Of course, those secrets are now history and important to disclose because of their threats to mankind. Nonetheless, I shall restrict myself to sharing information that has already (to the best of my knowledge) been revealed at some level. Physicians are forbidden by the Hippocratic Oath to use their professional knowledge in the service of harm; therefore, in its chemical and biological warfare programs, the Army cleverly utilized veterinarians, who have similar training but do not take the Oath. (There were, however, military physicians who disregarded it.) The incapacitating agents being studied and developed were largely psychotomimetic compounds, such as LSD, that lead to temporary confusion and mental aberrations. It was suggested to me that involvement with testing of these agents was compatible with the Hippocratic Oath because if one could incapacitate and capture an enemy soldier, one wouldn't have to kill him. These substances, could thus be considered lifesaving. Full of curiosity, I bought the argument (which has some merit), but I now feel in retrospect that even my inconsequential involvement had been unethical. "Do no harm" is the first principal of medicine.

Incapacitating agents were given, often *en masse*, to volunteers. (Of course, volunteers were enticed by the prospect of extra leave, good assignments, and the possibility of a better future career in the Chemical Corps.) I saw a number of untoward reactions, usually transient. As a requirement of my own voluntary participation, I was given LSD myself on several occasions, which were interesting, though not particularly pleasurable or harmful experiences. On one occasion, a group of Nationalist Chinese (Taiwanese) officers were observing a large group of our officers under the influence. A group psychosis suddenly materialized. The Nationalist officers were suddenly perceived as Communist Chinese spies! They were violently assaulted by the American officers. My colleagues and I frantically called for the Military Police to help up pull them off the hapless Chinese.

I was ordered on temporary duty to Fort Lee, Virginia, just outside Washington, D.C., to observe the performance of high command officers who were to have LSD slipped into their coffee during an annual paper and pencil "war games" exercise. (LSD is tasteless, odorless, and potent in tiny amounts.) It had been decided that, in wartime, such agents would not likely be employed indiscriminately but, rather, in selective ways. I was to be disguised as an infantry colonel. No one of lower rank than a colonel participated in such games. It was mainly generals. (I thought I was a bit young, at 25, for such a disguise to work.) I refused to participate on the grounds that a military physician cannot be ordered to perform a medical procedure that he or she feels is inappropriate. I asserted that giving a potent psychotomimetic agent of unknown dose (some officers, no doubt, would drink more coffee than others) to uninformed subjects was highly dangerous and unethical. Thankfully, it was not done. (I heard a rumor that such an episode eventually took place.) My own refusal to obey orders in situations that I considered to be immoral made me more empathic in subsequent studies of Vietnam veterans.

I was sent to a top secret three-day-long group briefing on chemical and biological warfare at the Army's Chemical Corps research center in Ft. Dietrick, Maryland. I believe that I was the first psychiatrist ever to attend such a briefing. We were observed by both identified monitors and "plants", lest we abscond with any notes. On reporting in, I was greeted by a physician-colonel who startled me by jumping out of the second story window, shrieking, "Oh, a psychiatrist, I'm going to kill myself!" As an ex-paratrooper, he knew how to fall. This commanding officer physician would routinely leave a new cap on a flagpole for a month to weather properly before he would wear it. What was really striking was that he carried a polished human femur (thigh bone) as a swagger stick. (Shades of Dr. Strangelove!) His eccentricities certainly did not do much for my insecurities about the development of lethal chemical and biological agents. In an amount invisible to the naked eye, the latest cholinesterase-inhibiting nerve gas applied directly to the skin was sufficient to kill a horse from convulsions within a minute. Germs were being bred (before genetic engineering) for antibiotic resistance. Although precautions were strict, God forbid if such a germ were ever to get loose (intentionally or not). Unlike atomic weapons technology, the capacity for biological warfare could easily be achieved by any number of third world countries, as was revealed in the frightening case of Saddam Hussein's Iraq. I understand that Ft. Dietrick has been closed and its labs have been converted to peaceful purposes. I saw how, through the erection of psychological defenses and rationalizations, justification of the most perverse and dangerous sort of behavior that could take place.

After a couple of thwarted attempts at publishing my observations in the Army, I basically quit writing them down.

Actually, I was able to publish one paper based on my military experience. I had wondered how one might predict success or failure in basic training. Since I had developed an interest in early memories, I systematically asked young male and female soldiers about their very first memory, hoping to determine whether it would betray something of their basic character or lifestyle. A couple of years later, when I first joined the faculty at Stanford, I discovered that my colleague and friend George Burnell, of UCSF, had similar interests. We enlisted the aid of the remarkable Margaret Thayler Singer, a person who had harnessed an uncanny intuition as a scientific tool. Margaret is a former President of the American Psychosomatic Society. We provided her with the brief first memories of men and women who had either succeeded at basic training or been discharged during it. Margaret was able with incredible accuracy (one in 10,000 odds of doing so by chance) to predict who would succeed or fail.

In both success and failure groups, memories were indicative of important life themes, or basic characterological approaches to life stresses, as had been first suggested by Alfred Adler. (Adler was one of Freud's original disciples who broke away to form his own school of psychoanalytic thought.) The selection of memory by the ego (the portion of psyche performing adaptive and defensive functions) is critical. While in the Army, I found that lay persons could match earliest memories with recurrent dreams, since both contained such basic life themes. (About 20% of all people, whether "neurotic" or "healthy", report having recurrent dreams.) I sometimes still ask, "Tell me the very first thing you remember and the age you were at the time." If the memory is from over the age of five, I assume that there is a lot of repression, either as a result of being out of touch with one's feelings or because of very painful early trauma.

Just the other day, I was given the answer, "Being alone in a pretty blue room. I was about three. That room was where I was sent when my parents didn't want me around."

I commented to that person, whom I had never met before, "I wonder if you tend to be a loner and kind of sad, in part because you believe you won't be accepted if you don't meet others' expectations."

"Amazing. Right on!"

Well, I've always said that an amalgam of input leads to unpredictable output. There must have been some connection between the Army and psychoneuroimmunology!

CHAPTER II

THE FIRST STEP—THE BEGINNING OF MIND BODY

*When the minds of the people are closed and wisdom is
locked out, they remain tied to disease. Yet their feelings and
desires should be investigated and made known,
their wishes and ideas should be followed; and then it
becomes apparent that those who have attained spirit and
energy are flourishing and prosperous, while those perish
who lose their spirit and energy.*

Huang Ti
(The Yellow Emperor; 2697 BC-2597 BC)

How was I to establish an academic career when I got out of the Army? The Chief of Research at Langley Porter, "Noch" Callaway suggested that I apply for a U.S. Public Health Service Career Teacher award, a two-year fellowship for post-residency training in academic medicine that would enable me to return to UCSF. I managed to get one of two psychiatry fellowships given that year. What a break! I could resume work with Jeffrey, and now Motoe, and I would have the opportunity to teach residents and medical students. The most amazing part of the deal was that the fellowship would largely pay for my own psychoanalysis because, in those days, personal therapy was still considered important training for a psychiatrist. (I wish it still were.) In addition, the fellowship would give me the invaluable opportunity to treat two patients three times a week under the supervision of a training analyst.

It might be timely to editorialize on my ambivalence toward psychoanalysis. For a couple of decades following World War II, academic psychiatry was dominated by psychoanalysis, and one could not achieve prominence in that area without a psychoanalytic background. (Psychoanalytic training was then restricted to physicians in the United States and was virtually a prerequisite for chairmanship of a university department of psychiatry.) Therefore, the discipline of psychiatry, which has major biological roots as a medical specialty, has largely been rooted in the psychology of the unconscious. In contrast, the field of psychology, with its foundation in learning theory, has focused primarily on behavior. Sigmund Freud, founder of psychoanalysis, was a neurologist by training and started off as a "biologist of the mind". He wisely abandoned his Project for a Scientific Psychology early in the century when he realized that the methodology of the day wasn't up to understanding the biology of thought and emotion. He knew he had to stick to the *psychology* of psychopathology. Still, he was much influenced by Nineteenth Century physics (repression, drive, etc., are quite hydraulic concepts) but, unfortunately, not by anthropology and sociology. I often wonder how Freud's genius would have dealt with neurotransmitters, neuropeptides, PET scans, and the like. Freud changed his ideas quite fundamentally on a number of occasions; however, his followers were not free to do so—as Adler, Jung, Rank, and others found out. Perhaps all the attacks on psychoanalysis from the outside, particularly by the medical profession, necessitated the "closing of ranks" and a religious-like adherence to dogma that has worsened since Freud's death because since then there has not been any giant to make changes from within. Nonetheless, major strides have occurred in two areas of psychodynamic psychiatry: ego psychology (Anna Freud, Hartmann, Kris, Lowenstein, Erikson) and object relations theory (Kohut, Kernberg).

It seems important to differentiate among 1) fundamental psychoanalytic principles (in contrast to the endless discourse that has filled psychoanalytic journals like Talmudic commentaries for decades),

2) psychoanalysis as a method of treatment for mental disorders, 3) psychoanalytic concepts as applied to psychobiological research, 4) the institution of psychoanalysis, and 5) psychoanalysts themselves. I am most comfortable with the first of these, psychoanalytic principles, and wish that more contemporary psychiatrists were. The unconscious, defenses, resistance (avoidance of issues that might lead to the awareness of painful unconscious material), and transference (transfer of feelings and attitudes about a formerly significant person to a current figure in one's life, particularly the therapist) seem to encompass the bread and butter of all but superficial and supportive psychotherapies—which, while not necessarily leading to conflict resolution, can still be helpful. At a recent psychoanalytic meeting, an elderly training psychoanalyst presented results from his follow-up of psychoanalyst trainees, who had been analyzed by him as part of their training process and who were now practicing psychiatrists. He had asked them to comment on key insights during treatment, key interpretations, major areas of repression, problems in working through particular conflicts, issues of the nature of transference, whether analysis had been beneficial, and what particular aspect of it had been most helpful. Remarkably, the psychiatrists had *not* been able to recount specifics from their therapy. Virtually all of them had found analysis helpful (as had I), and what they had found most helpful was their *relationship* with the therapist. It is eye-opening to discover the weight carried by the relationship with the therapist, even in classical analysis where the therapist attempts to be neutral.

The typical psychoanalytic process of treatment involves four sessions per week for a number of years. Fortunately, most neuroses (in contrast to some problems of character structure) do not require such heroic (and expensive) methods for cure. And how does insight cure? Insight may be essential to achieving the nondistorted (nontransferential) perception of others (especially the therapist) in order to make possible a "correct*ive* emotional experience". I maintain that insight for its own sake is desirable, especially for psychotherapists; however, I believe that insight must actively be *used* to bring about change. Freud himself said that he could assure more self awareness but not necessarily cure. I also feel that contemporary psychobiological research could benefit from a greater understanding of unconscious conflict but not in the symptom-symbolic way of early psychosomatic medicine. For example, I do not believe that the immunologically-related inflammatory bowel disease, ulcerative colitis, is a result of repeatedly getting rid of ("defecating out") the ambivalently regarded mother. I do believe, however, that *unconscious* conflicts can increase vulnerability to disease. To jump the gun a bit, Rudy Moos and I postulated that rheumatoid arthritics tended to be either very dependent or (more often) very independent, in contrast to a healthy control group. In other words, arthritics (and patients with other autoimmune diseases) seem to have unconscious *conflict* about their dependency needs, which they usually deny by hyperindependence (for example, never asking for favors). (If one were to average the test scores of the rheumatoid arthritics, they would look identical to the control group *vis-à-vis* dependency and these striking differences would be missed.)

Institutionally, psychoanalysis differs little from other organization establishments in its initiation rites and low tolerance for deviation from group norms. In regard to psychoanalysts themselves, I might paraphrase my subsequent colleague and friend, psychoanalyst, L Jolyon (Jolly) West, in saying that psychoanalysts are just like anybody else, only more so.

In my father's work, I became aware of the importance of the intangible "human factor", particularly humor, in therapy. One evening, Dad was in his study at home seeing a patient who continually sought to elicit reactions in others. Unable to get a rise from Dad, he escalated the stakes by finally threatening, "I'm going downstairs right now to rape your wife, and what are *you* going to do?"

Dad calmly replied, "I'm afraid I'm going to have to charge you for an extra visit." Laughter ensued, and insight was facilitated.

Although it may not have resolved all of my personal conflicts, my psychoanalytic background actually enhanced my research. Anxious to continue research on psychological factors in the onset and course of rheumatoid arthritis and other autoimmune diseases, I restored contact with the Rheumatic Disease Group when I became a fellow at UCSF, only to find that they had taken on a psychologist, Rudolf Moos, who had similar ideas. After a (surprisingly little) bit of initial tension over "turf," we decided to join forces. Thus, began the first of my few cherished long-term collaborations. Rudy Moos is gifted. He is quiet, intense, somewhat introverted, open-minded, and critical-thinking. Moreover, he was a good balance for me in his hypercautiousness and conservatism. He brought strength to our team in the areas of psychological testing, statistics, and research design.

A little side experiment that set the stage for my work with Rudy was an animal study that I did at UCSF with experimental psychologist, George Stone (and Jeff Fessel). Remember that arthritics were commonly described in literature as physically hyperactive, "on the go", sports-minded, and continually busy. Based on Dad's idea of arthritis as stemming from "frustration of motility", I wondered if curtailing activity in rats trained to be hyperactive would cause them to develop arthritis. We trained young rats to be hyperactive by giving them food rewards for activity wheel performance over a period of two months. Then, the wheel was simply locked (although the rats could still enter it), and the rats were fed without having to work for their meals. At this point, they became noticeably less adventuresome and more apprehensive. Although they looked unhappy to me, they didn't get arthritis. Oh well.

Serendipity struck. It was winter, and a window had been left open in the animal room, letting in a cool breeze. I noted that only the experimental animals (frustrated runners) near the window, had cold, blue-tinged paws, and this condition persisted for a while after they were moved to a warmer part of the room. This phenomenon was reminiscent of Raynaud's syndrome: excessive and persistent vasoconstriction in response to cold, commonly associated with autoimmune connective tissue diseases such as rheumatoid arthritis, scleroderma, and lupus. (Raynaud's *disease* occurs when the constriction is maintained, and tissue changes ensue.) Many have considered Raynaud's to be psychosomatic and precipitated by psychological stress. We decided to see if we could replicate the condition by placing *all* the rats in the refrigerator for one to two hours. After cold stress, only the motility frustrated rats had prolonged lower paw temperatures (as determined by thermocouple)—particularly when they had been frustrated for longer periods of time prior to refrigeration. We had experimentally produced a psychosomatic phenomenon in rats! Perhaps the rats would have developed overt arthritis if they had been primed with a very low dose of adjuvant (an immune-enhancing mixture of dead tuberculosis bacilli and oil that, in high doses, can produce rheumatoid arthritis-like joint disease in rats). (As much as I have wanted to do that experiment, I have never gotten around to it, nor has anyone else to whom I have suggested it.) We were delighted that the vascular disease journal, *Angiology*, published the paper. (I still wish more mainstream medical journals would publish relevant psychologically-oriented work.) I learned that it pays to be observant and that research doesn't always produce the outcome one expects.

I also want to mention a prescient but hardly-noticed research project that Rudy and I did with biochemist Alvin Halevy that same first year. Al had perfected a method of determining whole-blood (containing cellular elements, unlike serum or plasma) serotonin, a major brain neurotransmitter. About 95% of whole blood serotonin is found within the platelets, the cellular clotting elements of blood; 5% resides within plasma, the clear liquid portion of blood. We found that the severity of psychopathology in hospitalized psychiatric patients (schizophrenics, manic-depressives, and others) was correlated with the degree of *reduction* in whole blood serotonin. Since it is known that little, if any, serotonin passes between blood and brain because of the blood-brain barrier (especially tight blood vessel walls in the brain), critics had argued that platelet serotonin was irrelevant to brain metabolism, and, thus, to mental illness. Recall that whole blood serotonin is virtually synonymous with platelet serotonin. It is *now* known that what goes on in blood cellular elements (particularly, as psychoneuroimmunology has shown, in lymphocytes) may reflect what is going on biochemically in the brain. Recently, it has been found that patients with chronic physical pain or ongoing psychological distress of post-traumatic stress disorder (PTSD) have low levels of platelet serotonin. Low levels of blood serotonin are associated with irritability in humans; low serotonin is associated with reduced levels of affiliative, friendly behaviors and low dominance status in monkeys. This early work on platelet serotonin and psychopathology certainly anticipated my forthcoming conclusions that the body is not actually *compartmentalized* into autonomous systems (for example, clotting, nervous, immune).

Rudy and I sought to improve upon the limitations of traditional psychosomatic research. The generalizability of most studies was typically hampered by 1) insufficient information about patient characteristics, 2) overemphasis on measuring negative personality traits, 3) a circumscribed view of psychological conflict (not allowing for the possibility that it might manifest in different, even opposite, ways), 4) inadequate control groups, and 5) incongruous methods and theoretical orientations. We used experimenters representing psychoanalytic and behavioral orientations; we used carefully matched control groups (for example, same-sexed, nearest-aged siblings, which automatically controls for age, sex, socioeconomic status, family background, and so forth); we specifically tested for the expression of personality characteristics in radically different ways; we assessed personality by various means [that is, by the standardized Minnesota Multiphasic Personality Inventory (MMPI), another questionnaire specifically designed to assess situational behaviors, a semistructured interview, and role-play]. We also related psychological factors to blood tests and not just to disease (presaging psychoneuroimmunology).

Rudy had reviewed over 80 studies that reported psychological data on a total of over 5,000 patients with rheumatoid arthritis. Almost without exception, the investigators agreed that emotional factors were very important in the onset or course of the disease. We wrote down on little slips of paper any personality characteristics that were agreed upon by at least two investigators, yielding 140 slips in all. It was largely through these slips (which we sorted by means of the "Q-sort" technique) that we derived 19 scales of personality traits with extremes at either end:

1. Dependency vs. denial of dependency (hyperindependence)
2. Physical activity vs. motor inhibition
3. Duty, conscientiousness vs. lackadaisicalness
4. Compulsivity, perfectionism vs. disorderliness, slovenliness
5. Compliance, subservience vs. defiance
6. Bound, controlled, or repressed affect vs. free or impulsive affect
7. Masochism, self-sacrifice, denial of hostility vs. sadism
8. Nervousness, restlessness vs. calm, tranquillity
9. Reserved, introverted vs. outgoing, extroverted
10. Depression vs. elation
11. Conservatism, security vs. boldness, willingness to take risks
12. Overconcern about looks, impression vs. unconcern about appearance
13. Controlling, demanding vs. seeking control, understanding
14. Contrasexual identification vs. isosexual identification
15. Sensitivity (especially to others' anger) vs. insensitivity
16. Busyness vs. idleness
17. Emotional lability vs. emotional stability
18. Feels others' needs as demands, feels pressured vs. feels free of demands and pressures
19. Obliviousness vs. distractibility

Trying to hone in on the key dimensions related to rheumatoid arthritis, we compared the personality characteristics of sixteen female rheumatoid arthritics and their closest-aged, same-sexed, healthy siblings. Each subject was given the 556-item MMPI and a specifically constructed personality test describing scenarios expected to elicit telltale behavior in rheumatoid arthritics. In addition, the participants were given a 45-minute, semistructured, tape-recorded interview (independently evaluated by two raters) that included a short psychodrama (role-play) aimed at measuring assertiveness and expression of anger. The MMPI scores of our participants were compared against numerous scales. The nine *standard* scales (by which the test was originally scored) were those empirically derived by having administered the test to large groups of particular types of individuals, such as schizophrenics. These scales would reflect how such specific groups would answer the questions. The 113 *published* scales were scales that other investigators had empirically derived from their research using the test. Our 11 *rationally derived* scales were made up of individual MMPI items which we selected on the basis of their presumed relevance to the key personality dimensions of rheumatoid arthritics that we had outlined as a result of our literature review. Finally, we checked our participants' test scores against the three validation scales designed to identify lying. Arthritics scored significantly higher than their siblings in MMPI scales reflecting physical symptoms, depression, apathy, lack of motivation, anxiety, masochism, overcompliance, self-alienation, and psychological rigidity. Using combined interview and MMPI scores, rheumatoid arthritics showed the strongest differences in the dimensions of compliance/subservience, nervousness/restlessness, depression, and sensitivity (to anger). In addition, arthritics scored significantly higher in the areas of masochism/self-sacrifice and bound/repressed affect on the situation-specific personality test. Our data suggested that underlying characteristics were manifested in different or opposite ways.

In the interviews, patients tended to describe themselves as having always been nervous, tense, worried, struggling, depressed, moody, high-strung, and easily upset; whereas, siblings described themselves as sociable, active, constantly busy, affable, conscientious, and productive. Patients and siblings agreed closely with each others' assessments. The arthritics demonstrated more masochism, self-sacrifice, and denial of hostility in the psychodrama, in their descriptions of their marriage relationships, and in their responses to the question, "Tell me the last time you got angry." The last time they were angry was invariably a longer time ago than their siblings last were angry. Although parents were described in similar terms, patients struggled more with overstrictness on the part of their fathers and feelings of rejection by their mothers. Their mothers were often self-sacrificing martyrs who had unintentionally contributed to the patients' guilt about tending to their own needs. Unlike their sisters, whose marriages were average and reasonably happy, the arthritics tended to label their marriages as extremely good or bad. Husbands of female arthritics were typically either saintly, faultless paragons of virtue ("so good to me it's pathetic"), or mean and abusive but tolerated. The patients' unhappy marriages lasted for a considerable length of time (up to 27 years), in part because of their unassertiveness and strongly masochistic, self-sacrificing behavior. Interestingly, all siblings admitted fighting with their husbands, while over three quarters of the arthritics claimed never having argued with their husbands—even in the worst of marital conditions. Although uncontrolled for similar events in the lives of their sisters, almost every patient linked the development of arthritis with some acute or chronic stress situation. One patient was forced to move from one town to another against her strong wishes; another had a traumatic experience associated with surgery; a third developed arthritis during a year in which her father had a stroke, her brother-in-law passed away, her mother-in-law (whom she did not care for) came to live with her, and her house caught fire; still another needed to take care of her mentally ill husband for three years.

In the role-play psychodrama that we used to test assertiveness, I portrayed a nasty, unreasonable department store manager who refused to give a refund on a defective, recently purchased, and warrantied small appliance. In *every* case, the sibling was more assertive than the arthritic. Patients tended to give in quickly, remaining polite and in control the whole time. "It's certainly not fair, but I guess I'm stuck with it," was their typical response. The siblings threatened everything from calling the Better Business Bureau to filing a brief in small claims court. One sister actually pretended to hit me on the head with the defective steam iron!

A particular patient-sibling pair always stands out in my mind as being particularly illustrative. The sibling had the autoantibody rheumatoid factor, but was perfectly healthy. Both were attractive; the sister was gorgeous. The patient described herself as devoted to her perfect husband and three wonderful children. She then said, "Maybe I should tell you about my 'more masculine phase', before I got arthritis—a time I often recall with pleasure." The patient had been in the Air Force, the only woman at the time to have been an instructor in bomber engine repair. After leaving the service, she rushed into marriage, adopted the cliché (1960s) "a woman's place is in the home", and forced herself into the conventional social role of wife and mother. Despite her physical pain, she also served as caretaker to her elderly father, going to his home regularly to clean and cook. She was dutiful in those roles. It was during this period that she developed rheumatoid arthritis. In contrast, her sister (the winner of a major beauty pageant) had gotten pregnant at a young age and married the father despite reservations about him. Her husband was soon drafted and sent overseas during the Korean War. Upon his return, she discovered philandering. "He was out on his ass before he knew what hit him." At the age of 21, the sister began to compete internationally in a particularly difficult track event, achieving a U.S. women's record. At 26, she switched to a less strenuous sport on a professional level. She was fortunate enough to meet and fall in love with a man, also a pro in the same sport, with whom she wound up having a terrific marriage. They toured together doing what they both loved to do, and her son thrived. A disclosure was most revealing: "There is something about my sister and our background that I think you should know. I love my sister; she's a wonderful person, and we get along great, but I simply do not understand her. Our father sexually abused me as a child. I could almost swear he abused her, too, but she'll never talk about it. Now that our mother is dead—can you believe it—she goes over to his house to clean and cook food for his freezer. I hope the son of a bitch rots in Hell! When he dies, I'll dance on his grave!!" Similar? Different? Why arthritis in the patient? Why not arthritis in the rheumatoid factor positive sister?

Subsequent to the study of patient-sibling pairs, we gave the MMPI to a larger group of 49 female rheumatoid arthritics and 53 of their healthy female family members to see whether our previous findings could be generalized to a larger group of patients and a somewhat less closely matched control group. Our previous findings were essentially confirmed.

Rudy and I also attempted to correlate psychological variables with the *course* of rheumatoid arthritis in three studies. First, we compared people who were relatively incapacitated despite moderate objective evidence of disease (as shown by x-ray) versus those relatively functional in the face of severe disease. Second, we compared arthritics whose disease was progressing rapidly versus those with slowly progressing disease (galloping vs. creeping). Third, we compared patients with good versus poor response to treatment with injected gold salts. The results of all three studies were similar. The MMPI showed that patients doing less well were more physically symptomatic, psychologically distressed, isolated, controlling of impulses, dependent, and easily upset than their more functional counterparts. They also had lower ego strength (capacity for coping). The patients doing better maintained more adaptive coping skills and were more self-respecting and interested in people and events around them. Cause or effect?

Rudy and I needed a way to document that the personality traits relevant to the disease actually existed *prior* to the disease and not as a *result* of the disease. There is a tendency for rheumatoid arthritis to run in families (a genetic predisposition). Moreover, it is known that relatives who bear the rheumatoid factor in their blood sera ("FII" positive) are more likely to develop rheumatoid arthritis later in life than those who are FII negative. In what I consider prescient research, we compared the psychological characteristics of 14 *healthy*, FII *positive* relatives (about 80% of our sample of relatives) with 21 healthy FII *negative* relatives. No subject or investigator knew who was FII positive or negative. Who were the psychologically healthier? The FII *positives*, of course. The MMPI revealed that FII negatives represented a random sampling of the general population (like a comparison group of blood bank donors), some of whom were plagued by anxiety, alienation, lack of control, fear, guilt, poor self esteem, and psychiatric symptoms; thus, they ranged from very healthy to near crazy with most somewhere in-between. *All* FII positive relatives were in great psychological shape with good coping skills, a select group indeed. Although the FII positive relatives shared some characteristics in common with rheumatoid arthritics (such as inhibition of aggression and concern about appropriate social behavior), these psychological defenses appeared to be manifested in more functional ways. It seemed to us that psychological health was preserving physical health in the face of a genetic vulnerability. I would say to the FII positive relatives, "If, God forbid, some tragedy such as a loss of husband (wife) or child occurs, perhaps you should seek some special help to get through the stress as best as possible because there's a potential danger that you could develop rheumatoid arthritis."

One of the criticisms of psychoneuroimmunology, which to a degree has been made of psychosomatic medicine, is that the patient is being blamed for his or her own disease. Thus, the doctor is accused of making an already sick patient feel worse by virtue of guilt. I thoroughly disagree. I believe that psychoneuroimmunology should be *empowering* in view of its findings. There should be no place for panic, despair, and hopelessness. The patient has an active role in his or her own healing and is not merely a victim of disease. Moreover, psychological factors, such as difficulty in being nasty, can hardly be considered psychopathological. Sure, patients may need to rail at the nurse or express outrage to the doctor for treating them like an inanimate object or not treating them at all. Yet, should the more polite patient feel guilty about being so nice? Ridiculous!

Our paper demonstrating the role of emotional well-being in preserving physical health among those vulnerable to rheumatoid arthritis was reprinted in 1985, 20 years after its original publication, as a "classic in psychosomatic medicine". Rudy and I commented on our two-decade-old paper. According to our original model, integrated psychological functioning can prevent the process by which a predisposing biological agent would otherwise lead to overt illness. Although the core elements of this model remain valid, a new systems-oriented framework holds that biology, stressors, mode and success of coping, and social context are all complexly involved in health and illness. According to this logic, stressful social forces (such as chronic marital and job strain) can provoke depression or anxiety and thereby depress components of the immune system, increasing the risk of physical illness. Conversely, psychological cohesion (comprehensibility, manageability, and meaningfulness, according to Aaron

Antonovsky) and social support may buffer stress by lessening resultant *distress*. Lack of distress allows optimal functioning of the nervous and neuroendocrine systems, which in turn permits optimal immune functioning and preservation of health. (By emphasizing the active role of the individual in the development, management, and prevention of illness, behavioral medicine has taken a valuable step beyond the biomedical model. As a field, however, it has tended to neglect psychodynamic factors, limiting itself to a somewhat restricted view of coping processes and behavior.) A *truly* psychosomatic or biopsychosocial perspective for *all* disease not only can help eliminate now-untenable mind-body dualism but also can lead to the cross-disciplinary collaboration necessary to clarify the ways in which biological, personal, and contextual factors affect each other.

By 1963-64, pieces of a puzzle were beginning to come together. After doing together what I feel was some of the best psychosomatic research to date, Rudy and I realized that we had pushed the limits of the classical approach to the field. This approach, involving the *retrospective* or contemporaneous correlation of personality patterns or emotional conflicts with an organic disease, inevitably leads to several questions: Which came first, the disease or the personality trait/coping style pattern? Which came first, emotional distress or disease? Are the psychological characteristics and emotional states being accurately reported by the patients? Are the psychological parameters relevant to the disease in question? We saw the need for long-term, *predictive* studies of disease development in persons considered to be psychologically at risk as well as the need for studies of the *mechanisms* underlying psychosocial influences on pathophysiology (processes inducing disease or resulting in vulnerability to disease).

Such new approaches might resolve the longtime dispute within psychosomatics between those who believe that specific personality traits or conflicts are linked with particular diseases and those who hold that general distress can lead to diseases which are determined by constitutional vulnerability. My own bias has been toward the former point of view. Indeed, Rudy and I found that particular traits and coping patterns related to autoimmune disease (perhaps not only to rheumatoid arthritis) are different from those reported to be associated with coronary artery disease, the so-called "Type A" behavior pattern characterized by competitiveness, time urgency, and aggressiveness.

I puzzled over how the psychological factors we had observed must be transduced into physiological processes leading to rheumatoid arthritis and, possibly, to other autoimmune diseases. Suddenly, I had a "Eureka!" experience that *seemed* to make it all come together. I habitually review a lot of medical, psychiatric, and psychological journals to find links across the different perspectives. I had read in one of the medical journals that the prominent immunologist, Robert Good, linked autoimmunity not just to "excessive" immunity but to "immunological incompetence"; for instance, patients and mice with immune deficiency disorders have a high frequency of autoimmunity. Previously, I had learned of Frank Dixon's discovery that when a low amount of antibody was made in reaction to injected antigen, the result was formation of tissue-damaging antigen-antibody complexes (sometimes associated with autoimmunity). My mind was racing. Adrenocorticosteroid hormones suppress immunity. They are elevated by stress, as Hans Selye had originally shown and David Hamburg had demonstrated in major life stresses. Aha! Stress could be immunosuppressive via hypothalamic-pituitary-adrenal pathways, and steroid-induced immunosuppression could result in the formation of antigen-antibody complexes associated with autoimmune disease. The hypothalamic part of the brain (that regulates a variety of bodily functions) produces corticotropin-releasing hormone (CRH), which stimulates the pituitary gland to produce adrenocorticostimulating hormone (ACTH), which causes the adrenal glands to produce the hormone cortisol, which suppresses immunity. [Later, I proved myself at least partially wrong because stress could still suppress immunity in rats after removal of their adrenal glands. The rats were given injections of a steady dose of their adrenocorticosteroid hormone, corticosterone, to keep them healthy.] Moreover, schizophrenia is associated with immunologic abnormalities, as Jeffrey Fessel and I had found. Obviously, schizophrenia has to do with some sorts of brain dysfunction. The central nervous system *had* to be involved in immunity!

Next, came the clincher. I somehow ran across a brief abstract of a 1963 paper by Helen A. Korneva (soon to become a lifelong friend and colleague) and L. M. Khai of the Institute for Experimental Medicine (founded by Pavlov) in Leningrad (St. Petersburg), which reported that immunity could be virtually knocked out by small lesions in the hypothalamus. Simultaneously, Marvin Stein of the Mt. Sinai School of Medicine in New York prevented lethal anaphylaxis (allergic antigen-antibody reactions with massive release of histamine) by hypothalamic lesions in guinea pigs—a brilliant and foresighted experiment. It seemed to me only "right and proper" that the immune and central nervous systems be linked. Both serve functions of adaptation and defense. Both *relate the organism to the outside world* and differentiate friend from foe. Both have the property of memory and learn from experience (the immunologic basis for vaccinations). Both have a sense of self and nonself. Both have similar ways of going awry. In terms of the psyche, an inappropriate fearful reaction to something harmless, like a garter snake, is a phobia. A corresponding inappropriate reaction in the immune system is an allergy because, unlike germs, pollens are not intrinsically harmful. Either system can self-destruct. Psychoanalysis considers depression and suicide to be "retroflexed hostility". Autoimmunity is retroflexed immunological aggression. If the immune and central nervous systems have such similarities, perhaps they should have biological similarities as well. They should also be able to communicate with each other—the fundamental thesis of psychoneuroimmunology today. (More on this later.) In work at first as controversial as my own, the conceptual blockbuster Edwin Blalock, then at the University of Texas, Galveston, demonstrated that the *immune system* produces what were formerly thought of as only brain-regulated and produced substances: ACTH and beta-endorphin (a natural painkiller or opioid neuropeptide). Ed refers to the immune system as a "sensory organ", or sixth sense, that responds to stimuli that the five "regular" senses cannot detect (such as viruses and bacteria). The only one of the five senses that, like the immune system, detects on a molecular basis (and is closely related to emotional and memory centers of the brain) is the sense of smell.

Although we were not bold enough to be quite so explicit about our analogical thinking, in 1964 Rudy and I published "Emotions, Immunity, and Disease: A Speculative Theoretical Integration"—our last but most significant co-authored paper, which heralded the dawn of what I was soon to term "psychoimmunology". Our treatise began:

"Recent advances in immunology, clarification of the psychophysiology of stress, continued progress in the discovery of emotional factors in relation to physical disease, and the finding of apparent immunological disturbances in conjunction with mental illness lead to this attempt at a theoretical integration of the relation of stress, emotions, immunological dysfunction (especially autoimmunity), and disease, both physical and mental. At this stage, far more questions will be raised than answered. We come to this area of consideration via our own work on personality factors in rheumatoid arthritis, a disease with autoimmune features, and via collaboration with W. Jeffrey Fessel, who has done extensive work on serum protein abnormalities and autoimmunity in mental illness. This very speculative approach aims at encouraging the application of new basic medical concepts to psychiatry and at indirectly suggesting specific areas for future research. The time seems to be approaching when a meaningful synthesis of apparently disparate observations from basic and clinical medical and behavioral sciences may be possible and may serve a creative, heuristic purpose."

We also proposed, on the basis of growing evidence, that cancer could be immunologically resisted and that psychological factors might relate to its onset and course, as in autoimmune diseases. In regard to virally-induced tumors, Habel had theorized, "Perhaps the only way the mouse, naturally infected as an adult or infected with a small amount of virus as a newborn, can develop a polyoma tumor is by the *chance occurrence of some event* which temporarily reduces its immunologic competence at the proper time after viral transformation of normal cells to tumor cells [which are regarded as foreign by the immune system]." Could stress be the "event"? On the basis of Rorschach (ink blot) testing, Klopfer had found that rapidly metastasizing cancer patients were distressed and noncommunicative of that distress (that is, suppressed, not repressed), while unusually long-survivors of metastatic disease were either mature, calm, and accepting individuals or those able to avoid distress by "don't care" denial (that is, successfully repressed). We concluded in our paper that: "Relative immunologic incompetence, thus, may be both psychogenic and pathogenic . . ."

Eager to validate our theory, I declared, "Rudy, we've got to start a lab where we stress animals to see if we can suppress immunity. Then immunologists will be forced to believe that the brain has something to do with immunity, and clinicians will be convinced that feelings are important in resistance to disease. We'll call it the 'Psychoimmunology Laboratory'."

"Sorry, George, I'm just not into rats." Rudy wished me well. Choosing clinical over experimental psychology, he became a pioneer in social ecology (how environments elicit behaviors). He has developed psychological tests for social settings—hospitals, schools, jails, the workplace. Knowing both the personality "push" and the environmental "pull" for particular behaviors, one could accurately predict behavior. Although Rudy's creativity expressed itself in a very different way after 1964 (for which he became well-known), I feel that he also deserves credit for the genesis of psychoneuroimmunology. I got a new lab at the Stanford-affiliated Palo Alto Veterans Administration (VA) Hospital on campus and posted a sign next to the door: "Psychoimmunology Laboratory". Thus, began a new field.

CHAPTER III

THE GESTATION AND
BIRTH OF
PSYCHONEUROIMMUNOLOGY

Psyche and body, I suggest,
react sympathetically upon each other.
A change in the state of the psyche produces a change in the
structure of the body and, conversely, a change in the
structure of the body produces a change
in the state of the psyche.

Aristotle

I got the Psychoimmunology Laboratory, but quickly realized thatI didn't know anything about immunology. Why did I remember so little about the subject from medical school? Years later, I found a box packed with old textbooks. Looking up "lymphocyte" in my old microbiology text, there was a single sentence: "The function of the lymphocyte is unknown." Devoid of research funds, yet eager to begin my work, I set up some experiments that involved subjecting rats to stress and recruited my first lab assistant—a psychiatric patient at the VA needing "occupational therapy". I couldn't get any VA or National Institutes of Health (NIH) grants because not only was the idea of a relationship between stress and immunity viewed as "far out" (after all, the immune system was considered to be autonomous) but also I had no preliminary data to support my hypothesis. My assistant, Abel, had suffered a psychotic break while studying for his Ph.D. in immunology at Stanford and was now in partial recovery, living at a halfway house-type unit at the Menlo Park Division of the VA Hospital. This arrangement seemed mutually beneficial because Abel, not my own patient, could prepare for returning to the job market or graduate school, and I could get free help. My initial experiments were going amazingly well until one evening when I discovered Abel "dry labbing" (making up results). He was falsifying some data to please me. I was most chagrined and, although probably some of the data were okay, had to throw everything out—essentially wasting my first six months in the lab. I figured that as long as I was starting over, I should learn more about immunology. I got permission to sit in on the graduate course in immunology from Sydney (Sid) Raffel, the Chair of Stanford's Department of Microbiology and Immunology and a former medical school teacher of mine. I learned a lot but not about anything of use to me at the lab "bench". I needed techniques that I could use to evaluate aspects of the immune system in experimentally manipulated animals. So, I started approaching various immunologists about the possibility of learning some techniques in their labs.

The responses I got from immunologists, including those at Stanford other than Sid, were negative; however, I was invited to the prestigious Scripps Medical Institute and Research Foundation in La Jolla (near San Diego) by Frank Dixon, head of the Immunology Department. Dixon was a relatively young, yet distinguished, scientist who had investigated the pathological significance of antigen-antibody complexes—an area of study which bore some relevance to my work in autoimmunity. Despite his reputation for toughness, I found him to be kind and supportive.

I was assigned to work with Richard Dutton, who had co-developed (with Bob Mishel, brother of a med school classmate) a test tube (*in vitro*) technique simulating immune response in the body (*in vivo*). In this technique, one immunizes an animal with an antigen (a substance which will trigger an immune response) such as bovine serum albumin (blood proteins from a cow) and then removes the lymphocytes from its spleen. (Later, lymphocytes from peripheral blood could be used.) The same antigen is then added to an *in vitro* culture of the splenic lymphocytes. The lymphocytes responsive to that specific antigen would be stimulated to transform into immature blast cells capable of dividing (blastogenesis) and, thus, multiplying of that specific clone (identically responding group) of cells. This process represents a secondary ("recall" or "booster") antigen response. The antigen-specific technique had not been fully perfected, but it was working quite well in Dutton's lab.

[Most researchers in psychoneuroimmunology have subsequently utilized a set of compounds called mitogens to activate immune responses as a way of measuring the competence of a category of immune cells. Mitogens, generally plant-derived substances of a class called lectins, act as "super-antigens" that nonspecifically stimulate all clones of lymphocytes. Phytohemagglutinin (PHA) and concanavalin A (conA) are two mitogens that stimulate all T cells to proliferate. The mitogen pokeweed (PWM) stimulates mainly B cell clones. Another current nonspecific *in vitro* stimulant of lymphocyte blastogenesis is anti-T cell antibody, but our own work does not find it advantageous in human psychoneuroimmunologic research. Initially, I had thought that the overly powerful and nonspecific nature of mitogens would override any subtle effects of experience on immunity, but that proved wrong. The sensitivity of the antigen-specific technique may prove to be preferable in future.]

After a week of struggling to learn the technique at Scripps, I had a medical student, Philip Matin, come down from my lab to join me. I was certain that he would be much better than I at picking up the technique. Phil had a master's degree in physics and had been putting himself through medical school by scholarships, loans, and other means. At that time, Stanford had a wonderful system whereby medical students who worked up to half time in a research lab during their clinical years paid only half tuition. Moreover, there was no charge to researchers for the services of the students. I was particularly fortunate to have Phil in my lab because of his prior lab experience in physics. The blastogenesis test for lymphocyte activity that I was trying to learn involved the uptake of tritiated thymidine. (Tritium is a radioactive three-atom form of hydrogen that is taken up like regular hydrogen molecules when the cells grow. The absorption of tritium by the cells can be counted in a gamma radiation counter, and the amount of cellular growth can then be quantified.) Phil was familiar with radioactive techniques. I, on the other hand, was a klutz in the lab and had a penchant for spilling radioactive materials, sometimes flunking university inspections for lab contamination and having to submit to decontamination procedures. We supposedly learned this technique, but to my disappointment, we could never get it going properly. We had a confounding problem of culture contamination because Stanford was constructing a large series of new labs, including primate facilities, in the building where my lab was located at the VA, and the remodeling produced a lot of dust. Much time was wasted in struggling to set up the technique that we had tried to learn at Scripps. I needed some new techniques *and* some research funds.

Ironically, it was through bemoaning to my father the impossibility of getting grants for novel proposals, without having substantiating evidence, that I was able to get a bit of money privately. (One can get government money for *documentation* more easily than for true *experimentation*, the testing of novel hypotheses when the answer may be negative but interesting nonetheless.) Dad approached a wealthy former patient who had benefited greatly from psychoanalytic therapy and had established a rather large private foundation. I applied to the foundation and was granted some annual support, with which I was ultimately able to produce data that, in turn, enabled me to obtain research grants from the NIH. This experience led me to believe that *private* support is essential to the scientific process. The "peer review" system of the NIH is basically fair, but because of increasing demand for limited resources it is extremely conservative in its selections. European research funding, based more on institutional rather than individual ("entrepreneurial") grants, is less fair and more subject to authoritarian and political (institute director) control, but is sometimes more innovative *if* the institution lets its own good investigators have the freedom to test their own creative ideas. Eventually, my wife and I established a foundation (The Fund for

Psychoneuroimmunology) hoping to provide modest sums for young investigators, who do not have the necessary track record to obtain federal funding, and to allow a few gifted researchers to take some low probability, high gain research chances.

So there I was with the funds, but I was still in a quandary over where to get help in setting up appropriate immunology lab techniques that I could manage on my own. No immunologist in those days was interested in utilizing his or her lab to collaborate on stress research, so I needed my own lab. In desperation, I asked myself, "Who is the greatest immunologist in the world?" Perhaps that person would be more open-minded than most. Fortunately, for what turned out to be the field of psychoneuroimmunology, such was the case.

That immunologist was Sir MacFarlane Burnet, the recently retired but still active former Director of the Walter and Eliza Hall Institute of Medical Research in Australia—the greatest center of immunologic research in the world. Sir MacFarlane had won a Nobel Prize for his radical clonal selection theory of antibody formation, which stated that there were many hundreds of thousands or millions of specific preprogrammed cells triggered to replicate by encounters with a specific antigen. Prior theory had been that antigen served as a template for the production of antibodies that were then "stamped out" by plasma cells (the instructional theory). Sir MacFarlane's theory was controversial because of the incomprehensibility of so many genes within DNA in order to control production of so many different proteins. (It is now known that *combinations* of several genes enable antibodies to be produced in such varied specific types.) Sir MacFarlane's research was remarkably heuristic in that it spawned a whole new era of molecular immunology.

I wrote to Sir MacFarlane, who knew nothing of me, and told him of my ideas and my dilemma. I promptly received a most gracious letter in which he said that although he was skeptical about my ideas, particularly about the role of the central nervous system in regulating immunity, the concepts were nonetheless intriguing, and he would be interested in discussing these ideas with me. He also offered assistance in learning appropriate immunologic lab techniques through his young successor Gustav Nossal, Director of the Hall Institute. I wasted no time in getting to Melbourne for conversations with the gracious "Sir Mac" and for invaluable help from the remarkable Gus (now "Sir Gustav") and his colleagues.

Gus spent every afternoon in his lab at the bench doing very delicate single cell work observing the production of antibodies by individual lymphocytes. Although he was working as a basic (laboratory "bench") scientist, he was also a trained physician. Once a week he would make rounds on the Clinical Research Unit to maintain his medical knowledge, to remind himself of the relevance of his research to medical problems, and to glean research ideas from not yet understood clinical cases. In my experience, great thinkers are not narrow people. Gus was also interested in literature, arts, and the humanities. Since his lovely wife had no interest in science whatsoever, they had a rule that upon entering his home, science was not to be mentioned. Most of their guests were artists, musicians, writers. However, both he and his wife were interested in psychiatry and knew little about it; thus, what to do when I visited?

I met virtually all the distinguished immunologists at the Hall Institute. There were two with whom I had particularly close contact. One was Ian Mackay, who headed the Clinical Research Unit. Ian had helped establish insulin-dependent diabetes as an autoimmune disease, in which the immune system attacks the beta, insulin-producing, cells in the islets of the pancreas. He was also investigating pernicious anemia as an autoimmune disease. Ian and I were intrigued with the question of whether psychological factors associated with "connective tissue" autoimmune diseases, like rheumatoid arthritis, scleroderma, and systemic lupus erythematosus, were also similar in gastrointestinal autoimmune diseases. I sent him a potpourri of psychological research materials that Rudy Moos and I had used with the idea of comparing the two groups of patients with different types of autoimmune diseases.

The other person with whom I had fruitful contact was Senga Whittingham. Senga (Agnes—her mother's name—spelled backwards) is a remarkable, quiet, attractive, brilliant, shy person. Senga was particularly interested in multiple sclerosis, another autoimmune disease. She was a world expert in the fluorescent antibody technique, which involves tagging an antibody with fluorescein. The antibody then attaches *in vitro* to the portion of the tissue that it attacks, and that part glows under a fluorescent (ultraviolet) microscope. I got Senga interested in Jeff Fessel's and my idea of schizophrenia as an autoimmune disease and convinced her to try to replicate the controversial work of Robert Heath, of Tulane University, from whom that idea had gained most impetus. She was unable to replicate his findings. Although Heath's *work* may have been deficient (some say fraudulent), his *ideas* are fascinating and may yet prove to have some validity. (A hypothesis that fails to be proved may not necessarily be wrong; as important as negative findings are, they may mean that the *approach* to proof of the hypothesis is wrong.) Heath had discovered an alleged protein, "taraxein", in the blood sera of schizophrenic patients. He claimed that taraxein, when injected(!) into monkeys or *human volunteers*, produced "crazy" behavior. When working with Jeffrey, I had written to Dr. Heath asking whether taraxein might be an autoantibody. He replied, "No, because it is a beta globulin." (Antibodies are gamma globulins; taraxein is now considered a gamma globulin.) Heath then used the fluorescent antibody technique allegedly to show that antibrain antibodies attach themselves to brain cells of the septal-basal-caudate region of the schizophrenic brain. (He created antibrain antibodies by injecting portions of human brain into sheep, which produced immunoglobulins against the human brain antigen. The sheep immunoglobulins were then injected into brains removed from schizophrenic patients at autopsy.) He inferred from this study that schizophrenia was in fact an autoimmune disorder stemming from (auto)antibodies against a unique antigen in the septal-basal-caudate region of the brain. Heath later claimed that injections of taraxein could produce the same sort of electroencephalographic (EEG) spike activity in the septal-basal-caudate region of monkeys as spontaneously occur in the septal region of schizophrenic patients, into whose brains he had placed depth electrodes! (Try to get that through a Committee for Protection of Human Subjects nowadays.)

The work attempting to show that *schizophrenia may be an autoimmune disease* has continued to this day. Similar, but difficult to evaluate, research has been done by Russian psychiatrists M.E. Vartanian and associates, including his wife Diana Orlovskaya. Dr. Vartanian was second, and then first, in command of Soviet psychiatry in the days of the hospitalization of political dissidents as "mentally ill". When I was in Fresno I got a telephone call from Dr. Orlovskaya (not knowing then that she was Vartanian's wife). "I should like to visit you to discuss your research on immunity and schizophrenia."

"I'd be glad to, but how can that be arranged?"

"I'll come to Fresno."

"You mean you can come on your own all the way to Fresno just to see me?"

"Yes."

"Then please do so, and my wife and I would be pleased to have you as our house guest."

While Diana was staying with us, and after I found out that her ability to travel was because she was Mrs. Vartanian, I gingerly brought up the topic of the hospitalized dissidents, promising not to quote her publicly. She queried, "Is it not true that the *content* of delusions, in contrast to their presence, is culturally determined?"

"Yes."

"Is it not true that many American grandiose paranoid schizophrenics believe they are Jesus Christ?"

"Well, not so many, but I have encountered a few Christs during my psychiatric career."

"The Soviet Union is an atheist, communist country and *our* paranoid schizophrenics have political delusions." Dr. Vartanian and associates later described so-called "sluggish schizophrenia", characterized by intact mental functions except for the presence of political delusions. Apparently, it only existed in the Soviet Union.

Years later, Dr. Vartanian traveled to Leningrad for the sole purpose of attending a dinner party given for me at the home of Helen Korneva when I was observing her latest, excellent work on the central nervous system and immunity at the Institute of Experimental

Medicine. I inquired, "You came because you are interested in Helen's work?" He replied, "No, I came to honor you because of your kindness to Diana." At a later date in Moscow, he told me that hospitalization of dissidents was a way to "protect" them from execution or imprisonment. I was proud of the stand of U.S. psychiatrists in pushing for the expulsion of Soviet psychiatrists from the World Psychiatric Organization. They, of course, regained membership as Russians after the fall of the Soviet Union in spite of the continued prominence of Dr. Vartanian (some of whose research, indeed, seems interesting). The issue of schizophrenia as an autoimmune disease is still being pursued at the University of Pittsburgh by Rohan Ganguli, Bruce Rabin, and associates.

Gus Nossal was perspicacious enough to realize that, given my level of laboratory know-how and intrinsic klutziness, I needed to learn a simple technique. He suggested that we use very small doses of a potent "novel" antigen (one to which an animal could never have been exposed and, therefore, to which it has not previously developed antibodies). In this way, there would be no confusion as to whether a particular immune response was primary or secondary (booster). I used flagellin, which is made of the flagelli, or the little beating "paddles", of a type of salmonella bacteria to which neither rodents or humans are generally exposed. This antigen was both expensive and in short supply; nonetheless, Gus generously kept me supplied throughout my studies of antibody formation. Now I had a lab technique that was doable.

Thus, began the flowering of the Psychoimmunology Laboratory. I had funding. I had a lab technique. And now I had a lab assistant, Suzanne Donohue, and medical student assistants, first J. Kersten Kraft, then Phillip Matin, who eventually made a number of contributions to nuclear medicine and became a faculty member at University of California, Davis. They were loads of fun. The lab atmosphere was lighthearted and relaxed; we could laugh about all the mistakes that we made. The lack of encouragement from elsewhere was compensated for by our collective sense of humor. Together we made many laboratory observations, some of which were never reported. For example, we found that when stressed animals were housed in the same room with unstressed animals, they would all exhibit stress responses. Therefore, we housed experimental and control animals in separate *quiet* (non-stressful) rooms. Many years later, it was discovered that a stressed animal transmits pheromones through the air via the olfactory system to induce a stress response in an unstressed animal.

Our little crew did the first two experiments in the field of PNI in the late '60s. The first paper was produced in collaboration with Seymour "Gig" Levine, a very distinguished psychoneuroendocrinologist, who once turned down a most internationally prestigious position in experimental psychology at Oxford. Gig had shown that the handling of neonatal rats changes their adult behavior *and endocrine* patterns. Newborn rats that were picked up and placed in a different environment, or given electric shocks, for three minutes daily until weaning at 21 days showed more adaptive behavior in adulthood when placed in new environments (that is, they defecated less, explored more freely, and habituated more quickly). They also showed a stronger and briefer adrenocorticosteroid hormone response to stress. From these studies, Gig concluded that stimulation in infancy may promote better psychobiological adaptation to unfamiliar environments in adulthood.

We did a similar study, reported in the British journal *Nature*, in which we gave neonatally handled vs. non-handled rats primary and secondary immunization with flagellin after they had grown to adulthood. The neonatally handled rats, which had been placed in a three-inch square box and gently stroked for three minutes a day before being returned to their nest, had better primary and secondary immune responses to the antigen (that is, they had more specific antibody to flagellin) than did the unhandled rat controls. It should be noted that after a rat pup has been briefly removed from its mother, it will receive excessive attention and nurturing upon return. In contradistinction, other scientists showed later that premature weaning at 19 days has the opposite effect—a lowered immune response in adulthood. A few years ago, George Vaillant conducted a 45-year follow-up study of a group of Harvard sophomore men who had been evaluated psychologically at age 20 in order to predict factors related to later mental and physical health. He found that the best predictor of the men's *physical* health at age 65 was the report at age 20 of having had a warm relationship with their parents. A good childhood is good for your health—even if you are a rat!

In our second study, we tested primary and secondary antibody responses to flagellin in rats subjected to three different kinds of daily stresses. One type of stress involved low-voltage electric shock delivered to the feet after an apprehension-inducing warning buzzer. The second mode of stress was produced by overcrowded housing conditions. The third form of stress consisted of being stranded on a small platform surrounded by water. This stress resulted in REM (rapid eye movement) sleep deprivation because muscles are inactivated during REM sleep, causing the rat to fall into the water and wake up. (Muscles relax during REM sleep to prevent acting out in dreams. Sleepwalking is caused by the failure of the muscles to be inactivated.) Only overcrowding stress reduced primary and secondary antibody responses, although REM deprivation reduced primary antibody response. [Perhaps the profound effect of overcrowding on immunity has teleological significance in terms of population regulation. Population density may produce a milieu of stress among animals (including humans?) resulting in lowered immunity, epidemics, and population reduction.] The peak primary antibody response of rats subjected to apprehension-electric shock stress was actually *higher* than that of the non-stressed control group. Thus, it was clear that different *forms* and *duration* of stress could have distinct effects on the immune system.

It quickly became apparent to me that I needed to collaborate with a sophisticated immunologist in order to access a *range* of tests for other aspects of immune function besides antibody formation. By now, I had obtained funding from the NIH and VA and had the wherewithal to support a basic scientist who would be willing to come to Stanford to collaborate with me. Through the aegis of Sid Raffel, who helped out once again, I was able to entice immunologist Alfred Amkraut, of the University of Oregon Primate Center, to work

with me. It took great courage for Alfred to be the first immunologist
to commit to PNI. (Now there are many.) Born in Germany to a
Jewish family who became refugees, he was reared in Bolivia and was
fluent in German, Spanish, Hebrew and English. After college and a
successful but boring episode with business, he came to Stanford for
his Ph.D. in immunology. Alfred relished the opportunity to return
to Stanford, where he was given a joint appointment as Assistant
Professor of Psychiatry and of Microbiology and Immunology. His
brilliance, competence, obsessive meticulousness, and conservatism
served us well in this controversial field because we never published
anything that hadn't been replicated in our laboratory three or four
times. (Twice seemed enough to me; I was wrong.) The downside of
Alfred's conservatism was that important observations were often buried
in a sentence or two within a paper, rather than being highlighted in
a separate report. (Nowadays, people do one research study and write
four or five papers based on it. We used to do four or five research
studies and write one article about it. Both seem improper, but I find
particularly offensive the contemporary emphasis on *numbers* rather than
quality of publication as the major criterion of academic promotion.)

We wanted to study the effects of stress on *cellular*, not only
humoral (antibody) immunity. Cellular (non-antibody) immunity is
responsible for graft and tumor rejection as well as the killing of
virus-infected cells. Therefore, the graft vs. host reaction presented a
good way of achieving our goal. In graft vs. host reactions, immunologically competent cells from the donor (graft) will attack cells from
the recipient (host). This phenomenon can occur in "allogenic" bone
marrow transplants, where the donor is not oneself or an identical
twin. To create a graft vs. host reaction in the lab, one crossbreeds two
inbred (genetically identical) strains of rats, producing an "F-1" hybrid, which has genes of both strains. Lymphocytes are taken from
the offspring and injected into the footpad of the parent. The part of
the lymphocyte (graft) bearing the genetic component from the *other*
parent will attack cells from the parent recipient (host). We discovered
that stress *reduced* or completely abrogated the graft vs. host reaction

chiefly through suppression of the host immune response, including production of substances that enhance graft vs. host reactions.

In light of Helen Korneva's discovery of *direct* regulation of immunity by the brain, I wished to visit her lab to see if her work was for real. (At the time, Soviet biological research was particularly suspect.) I applied for funds to travel to Leningrad under the new Soviet-U.S. scientific exchange program, but was turned down because psychiatry was "not included in the treaty". I wrote to the State department, "This work is immunology, not psychiatry." They wrote, "Sorry, but you are a psychiatrist." Not yet having found funding for the trip, it so happened that while returning from my semiannual ski trip to Aspen, I sat next to an Indian gentleman in the Vista Dome of the wonderful old California Zephyr train. We struck up a conversation. He was Minister of Railroads for India, and his orthodox Hindu brother, a physician and guru, held the only chair in traditional Hindu medicine (Ayurveda) in India at Benares Hindu University. Benares (also called Varanasi) is the holiest city in India, the site of the burning ghats where devout Hindus go to die, be cremated, and have their ashes scattered in the Ganges. Mr. Shukla was on his way to the Stanford Research Institute. I invited him to dinner at our home in Los Altos Hills. His thank you note from India stated that karma (fate) must have sat us together in the Vista Dome since we obviously had been soul mates in a previous incarnation, and karma would see to it that we would be together again in the shadow of the immortal Taj [Mahal]. Moreover, just to help karma along a bit, how would I like to come to India as guest of the Indian government and not only be able to visit him in New Delhi but also spend time with his brother in Benares learning something of Ayurveda?

Having had a long-standing interest in traditional systems of healing, for which our new research seemed to offer some possible explanations, I decided to take a detour from hard science and accept his invitation with the intent to continue on to Leningrad. After a short, pleasant stay in Delhi, I had a rare and meaningful experience in Benares. Harish Shukla, indeed, was a holy man, a healer. Harish's additional training in "modern" medicine had instilled in him the wish to prove some of the tenets of Ayurveda scientifically. Later (but well before Deepak Chopra), Harish and I wrote a paper on the relevance of Ayurveda to some contemporary ideas of "holistic medicine".

The basic writings of Ayurveda date back over 2,000 years. Among its very complex and systematized ideas, most of which seem contradictory to modern understandings of physiology, are some highly prescient concepts. These include "psychophysiological response specificity", namely that some people respond biologically differently from others. In Ayurveda, this concept is based both on body type (somatotype) *and* personality. Harish had demonstrated that one Ayurvedic type, associated with voluminous urination, actually *did* have deficient antidiuretic hormone responses to water deprivation. Moreover, ancient Ayurveda could readily be interpreted as embodying concepts of both natural and acquired immunity, along with the idea that resistance to disease could vary by both typology and experience, views most collegial with psychoneuroimmunology.

I asked to meet the Professor of Psychiatry, the sole member of the Department of Psychiatry and the only psychiatrist at the time for a population of several million. Well-trained in England, the Professor exclusively saw only rare violent paranoid schizophrenics on an outpatient basis; lesser cases of mental illness were too trivial. Since there were no *psychiatric* beds in the Benares Hindu University Hospital, I requested, therefore, to make *medical* rounds. Once was enough. The first patient, clearly moribund and wracked by coughing, was being propped up by his wife and surrounded by his children. The diagnosis was "septic [meningococcal] meningitis", a highly contagious disease. Soon, I observed the phlebotomist (blood drawer) using the same glass syringe *and* needle, which he wiped off with a bloody rag, on more that one patient. Several patients were expatriate American "hippies" with severe hepatitis, a viral disease very easily transmitted by blood. I felt I must speak out and blurted, "Please excuse me, but do you realize that the phlebotomist is using the same equipment on more than one patient?" The attending physician said, "Oh, you Americans are so technology-oriented!" (My experience lecturing at the University of New Delhi Medical School was quite different.)

I decided to fly to Leningrad to see Helen. When I eventually arrived in Leningrad, Helen Korneva could not recognize the "distinguished American scientist", who wearily emerged from the Aeroflot turboprop in an Afghanistan-obtained lamb fur (karakul) hat and gold-embroidered red vest. Helen's work was, indeed, for real. Her exciting and advanced brain-immunity work is still ongoing at the Institute of Experimental Medicine, where the world's only statue to an experimental animal—Pavlov's dog—is located. On my early trips to her laboratory, the oppressive atmosphere of the Communist state was omnipresent. Helen would only speak openly to me on nonscientific matters when walking on the street (however cold), certainly not in my government-provided chauffeured car. It was later that I realized Helen's courage and trust in promoting Viktor Klimenko (who later spent several months at UCLA) to the position of Assistant Director, Experimental Pathology Division. I didn't know then that Viktor's father was Jewish. Were Viktor to defect or apply for emigration to Israel, her career would have been ruined.

Back at the Psychoimmunology Lab, Alfred and I sent over to Leningrad a specially hired physiological psychologist, Phyllis Kaspar, to learn Helen's methods. I knew that I (the ultimate lab klutz) would never be able to execute the delicate placement of lesions in very tiny areas of the brain by use of a stereotaxic apparatus. Phyllis came through, and we were able to show that hypothalamic lesions affected the graft vs. host reaction—an example of an important but quite buried observation in our paper.

Alfred and I wanted to look at stress and tumor immunity. There is a type of connective tissue tumor that can be virally induced in mice called Moloney virus sarcoma. This tumor is normally resisted by the animal's immune system. Tumors grow, then regress with about 80% survival, while 20% of the animals develop widespread cancer and die. At the time, it was disputed as to whether virally-induced tumors existed in man, but it is now known that they do. Cervical carcinoma is associated with the human papilloma virus. Non-Hodgkin's lymphoma and nasopharyngeal carcinoma are related to the Epstein-Barr virus. Although it has never been shown in humans, mammary carcinoma (breast cancer) is virally related in mice and transmitted by mother's milk.

Our experiment required the use of females of an expensive in-bred strain of mice; therefore, I was disturbed to find that we were receiving damaged animals from the supplier. Some of the mice were marred with scabs, knicks, and cuts. We didn't want to use animals that might have been unhealthy or exposed to other stressors. Consequently, I called the supplier, expressing my dissatisfaction with his product. The person to whom I spoke said, "I'm terribly sorry. You must have accidentally gotten some fighters which we routinely try to destroy."

(Incredulously) "Do you mean that some of these genetically identical mice fight and some don't, particularly females?"

"That's correct."

"Can I come down and observe this for myself?"

"Yes."

I went to Gilroy (south of San Jose), where the breeding facility for these mice was located. Indeed, some of the mice fought, and others did not. (There are behavioral differences in genetically different strains of rodents, and in more recent years it has been shown that the behavioral differences in different *strains* can be accompanied by immune differences; however, these animals were all from the *same strain!*) I requested a regular supply of fighters and non-fighters so that in addition to studying the effects of a stressor and its timing on tumor growth, we could take into account behavioral factors as well.

We discovered that female mice subjected to three days of electric shock stress following virus inoculation displayed increased tumor size and mortality; whereas, those shocked for three days *prior* to virus exposure showed a *reduction* in tumor size. Moreover, we found that the spontaneous *fighters* developed *smaller* tumors and had a higher recovery rate. Our previous work had shown that electric shock did not alter the course of disease in males, but sex segregation had a damaging effect. This finding was confirmed. Apparently, not only *type* but also *timing* of stress can be a factor in the course of neoplastic (cancerous) disease.

A decade and a half later (without having read our papers), experimental (animal) psychologist Mark Laudenslager of the University of Colorado ran a series of experiments very similar to ours and came to the parallel conclusion that the *nature, duration, and timing* of the stressor in relation to the administration of antigen were all important factors in immune functioning. Also, in recent years at the UCSF, Lydia Temoshok, who had identified the relationship of psychological factors to physical markers associated with progression of malignant melanoma in humans, again showed that individual behavioral differences were relevant to cancer. She studied outbred (non-genetically identical) hamsters, in which behavioral differences might be expected, and found that the hamsters who were more socially interactive had less thick tumors that showed fewer mitotic figures (that is, less evidence of rapid tumor cell division) and greater lymphocyte response to the tumor. (I admire clinical researchers who attempt to carry human observations to experimental animal models.)

Alfred and I were also interested in the effect of stress on experimental autoimmune disease (since I had previously worked on human rheumatoid arthritis). If one injects adjuvant into rats, they develop an arthritis (particularly in the paws) that histologically resembles rheumatoid arthritis. It seemed logical that stress would *alleviate* the arthritic symptoms, since it elevates adrenocorticosteroid hormones, which are anti-inflammatory and used in the treatment of rheumatoid arthritis. We found, however, that group housing stress in male rats, with or without overcrowding, made the adjuvant-induced arthritis worse.

Wanting to take a closer look at the intermediary factors responsible for the effects of stress on specific elements of the immune system, I undertook a study of the effects of stress ` and adrenocorticosteroid hormone levels on interferon production in mice. The project was done in collaboration with Gig Levine and another outstanding member of the Stanford faculty, Thomas Merigan—one of the discoverers of interferon. Interferon (a cytokine) is a peptide, or small protein, made by various cells of the body but particularly by macrophages of the immune system. It not only has immune-regulating properties (poorly understood at that time), but also it can attack viruses directly and may play a defensive role against virus-induced tumors. (It is now used in the treatment of Kaposi's sarcoma in patients with AIDS.) Both stress and pharmacologic levels of adrenocorticosteroid hormone had been reported in the scientific literature to suppress interferon synthesis.

We measured interferon and corticosterone levels in mice six hours after injection with Newcastle Disease virus (NDV). Unexpectedly, we found that the stress of repeated random electric shocks preceded by a warning buzzer did not affect interferon production when it occurred after NDV inoculation, but stress significantly *enhanced* interferon production when it was given for five hours *prior* to viral exposure. Virus alone causes increases in corticosterone levels whether stress occurs before or after inoculation with virus. Since the administration of corticosterone did not alter interferon response, yet adrenal gland removal results in high interferon levels, we hypothesized that the increased interferon production associated with stress-preceded viral exposure may have been due to adrenal exhaustion from the chronic stressor. (This theory is analogous to Hans Selye's General Adaptation Syndrome "stage of exhaustion".) In other words, the viral challenge may not have been able to produce a maximal adrenal response that would have decreased interferon levels. Other studies, however, utilizing more modern methods of interferon measurement, have reported *decreased* interferon levels in response to different types of stressors. Our interferon research anteceded, by many years, any other studies of the effects of stress on cytokines. (Cytokines are peptides that transmit messages within and from the immune system.)

The work with rodents helped my conviction about the validity of psychoneuroimmunology in a personal way. I developed an allergy to rats, which I think reflected my distaste for working with them. Rats, intelligent animals, must have sensed my attitude because they kept biting me. I had such terrible bouts with hay fever that I would have to wrap moist towels around my mouth and nose to filter out the dander. Thinking that I might be better off, I began some experiments using mice. (Possible health advantages notwithstanding, the scientific advantage of working with mice is that mouse immunology is better understood than rat immunology; however, one cannot extract as much blood from mice.) Predictably, it wasn't long before I developed an allergy to mice as well. (This, of course, was a good excuse to palm off more of the animal work on my lab assistants.)

Resurrecting my old interest in schizophrenia and immunity, Alfred and I embarked on more studies of globulin abnormalities in schizophrenic patients. Since psychotropic drugs could interfere with immunity, we tried hard to locate drug-free schizophrenic patients. Fortunately, two-time Nobel Prize winner Linus Pauling, then at Stanford, had been able to arrange for a ward at nearby Agnews State Hospital where patients were given no medication but just vitamin C. It was a wild place because of the severely psychotic behavior of such patients. Dr. Pauling had begun his claims that vitamin C cures everything, including schizophrenia. Although his claims seemed farfetched at the time, a number of his ideas about antioxidants have since been validated but, unfortunately, not his ideas about schizophrenia. Dr. Pauling was so brilliant and charismatic that he nearly had *me* persuaded. I wanted to measure different classes of immunoglobulins in the patients; unlike neuroleptic (antipsychotic) drugs, I didn't think the vitamin C treatment would affect immunoglobulins much. Dr. Pauling agreed to give me access to his research unit. It turned out that immunoglobulin G (IgG), immunoglobulin A (IgA), and immunoglobulin M (IgM) levels were significantly elevated in these schizophrenic patients compared to normal controls. Furthermore, patients with lower levels of both IgG and IgA were more likely to show clinical improvement over the course of hospitalization.

Given the peculiar immunoglobulin profile of schizophrenics, I wondered if they would exhibit altered antibody responses upon encounter with an antigen. Because of the difficulty in getting permission from the human subjects protection committee to do a study exposing humans to an antigen to which they have never been exposed, like flagellin (even though it would present no danger or benefit), we chose instead to observe immune responses to tetanus booster injections in schizophrenic patients. Since tetanus immunizations had been a standard childhood event, and long-lasting immunity to tetanus was typical, we felt safe in assuming the relative homogeneity of the group's previous exposure to the toxoid vaccine. My Australian connections turned out to be helpful for this project. We sent blood sera to clinical immunologist Sydney Rubbo in Australia because his assay for tetanus antibodies was not only highly sensitive but also difficult to accomplish. We found no differences between schizophrenics and normal individuals in their immune responses to the tetanus toxoid injections; however, non-schizophrenic psychiatric patients showed a somewhat impaired immune reaction. Since most non-schizophrenic psychiatric inpatients suffer from depression, perhaps we had stumbled upon depression-induced immunosuppression without realizing it. Although immune responses to a novel antigen might have been more revealing, it was still worthwhile to report the negative results as we did. Lamentably, negative findings are hard to get published, but they are important for two reasons: they are often the outcome of a truly novel idea that may or may not be true (a genuine *hypothesis*); and they may spare someone else the disappointment of attempting to "reinvent the wheel".

Earlier research on abnormal immunoglobulins in schizophrenia, which I had published in conjunction with my colleagues at UCSF, revealed that many schizophrenic patients (and some other psychiatric patients as well) had particularly high levels of IgM. IgM appears first in response to initial antigenic stimulation (primary immune response), after which point IgG provides a more lasting immunity. We also knew that individuals with highly excessive levels of IgM can be treated with chlorambucil. The idea of using an immunosuppressive drug to treat psychiatric illness is both radical and problematic. Immunosuppressive drugs can render persons more susceptible to infection, although these drugs are used rather commonly to suppress autoimmune diseases and to prevent rejection of organ transplants. Bearing this in mind, and, of course, with approval of the human subjects protection committee, we gave *extremely* low doses of chlorambucil to some of the patients while others received a placebo. White blood cell counts were very carefully monitored to guard against drug-induced bone marrow suppression. Only one subject showed a marked drop in white blood cell count. For that individual, we broke the blind nature of the test (neither participants nor personnel knew who was taking the drug) and found that the patient had actually been on the *placebo*. There were no side effects from the extremely low doses of the drug; however, there were neither effects on schizophrenic illness nor IgM levels. We had selected patients with high levels of IgM on the presumption that they might be helped by a drug that would lower the levels. This negative finding may have been due to the fact that we used virtually homeopathic (tiny) doses.

As will be pointed out in the chapter on criminal behavior and violence, I took consulting jobs while running the Psychoimmunology Lab. One was with the University of Santa Clara, a Jesuit liberal arts college just south of Stanford. Originally, I was brought on as consultant to the Counseling Service headed by K. Michael Schmidt, Ph.D., and his associate, Jon Kangas, Ph.D. Although primarily a clinician, Mike was interested in doing some clinically relevant laboratory research. We explored the effects of restraint stress on the development of gastric ulcers in rats. We discovered that both vitamin E and, interestingly enough, *alcohol* helped prevent stress-induced ulcers. Alcohol increases gastric secretion, particularly hydrochloric acid, which is generally not beneficial for stomach lining; therefore, we speculated that the tranquilizing effects of alcohol must have buffered the stress effects. After all, the drunk rats seemed not to be bothered much by the restraint! This work anticipated later research of others showing that anti-anxiety drugs like ®Valiumä (diazepam) can block immunosuppressive effects of experimental stress in rats.

Mike's successor at the counseling service, Jon Kangas, and I shared an interest in *optimal* human functioning (in contrast to normal or normative functioning). We wrote a short paper on "The Psychology of the Strong Person" which was published in the Jesuit magazine, *America*. To our surprise, the Prentice-Hall Publishing Company saw the paper and invited us to expand it into a book entitled, *The Psychology of Strength.*

In our original article we listed the characteristics of the strong person:

He/she is relatively secure personally with "where s/he is at".

He/she is optimistic.

He/she is highly self-actualizing. Being relatively sure in his or her own basic needs for security, safety and esteem, s/he has moved toward fulfillment of maximal potentialities.

He/she validly sees him or herself as more productive than others.

He/she is flexible, and this flexibility is manifested by ease of movement among and completion of a variety of tasks.

He/she has less need than most persons for the approval of others.

In relationship to values, moral standards, and criteria for personal behavior, he or she is more inner-directed than other-directed.

He/she is tolerant of the weaknesses of others but often not of those in him or herself.

He/she is relatively unprogrammed by the past, that is, s/he has a great number of conflict-free areas that allow a greater range of choice and self-determination. S/he does not view the present through a "rearview mirror" or through "past-colored glasses".

He/she is relatively self-contained.

His/her self-esteem is internalized or "built-in".

He/she is comfortable in a variety of interpersonal encounters, shifting roles while maintaining personal identity and integrity.

He/she has less pressing need for the love of others.

He/she is not addicted to achievement *per se.*

He/she can delay gratification.

More people draw on his or her strength than he/she on theirs. People who are in contact with the strong person look up to, seek counsel from, and respect him or her.

His/her strength stems from a storehouse of mastered experience. This strength can be characterized as the sum of mastered experiences minus the sum of failures. S/he has had adequate opportunity for mastery, but challenges have not been overwhelming nor premature.

He/she tends to take for granted his or her strength.

He/she can focus and channel emotional and intellectual energies.

He/she is resilient in crises and has a command of a variety of coping strategies.

He/she is likely to see him or herself as a strong person.

A central point that we made was that strength can be looked at as the sum of one's mastered challenges minus the total of one's defeats. Each developmental phase presents its own challenges, the outcome of which determines the nature of "ego traits". Weakness ensues when life's challenges exceed the capacity of the individual to adapt or when an individual is somehow deprived of the opportunity to encounter necessary age appropriate challenges. For example, an abandoned five-year-old could not possibly meet his or her own needs for food and shelter and would be terribly damaged by the experience. On the other hand, an overprotected and indulged child would also become a weak adult because he or she would never learn how to deal with the inevitable hardships of life. This principle is true for the immune system as well. A perfectly healthy newborn animal that is placed in a germ-free environment until adulthood succumbs quickly to infection when removed from that environment because there have been no challenges to the immune system during development. We cautioned that every person, no matter how strong, has problems that require help and support; the strong person is often reluctant to break out of the caretaker mode and seek assistance. We also made the distinction between genuine strength and pseudo-strength, the latter represented by overachievers, "nice guys", martyrs, people with stable but narrow lifestyles, or rescuers (who derive vicarious satisfaction from identifying with the recipient). The strong person is easily recognized when adversity strikes. He or she tends to be highly principled, humanitarian, and drawn to helping and human service professions. Later in my career, I tested the theory that psychological strength contributes to health by evaluating a number of these characteristics in long-survivors of AIDS and healthy elderly persons. This work is described later.

I do not intend to write a history or review of

psychoneuroimmunology, but a few highlights are in order. What really put psycho-neuroimmunology "on the map" in the face of so much skepticism was the 1975 report of Bob Ader's and Nick Cohen's elegant experiments showing that immunosuppression could be conditioned by classical Pavlovian techniques. If saccharin *alone* could produce immunosuppression, after having been paired (conditioned) with the immunosuppressant drug cyclophosphamide, then the brain must be involved. Following conditioning, Bob showed that saccharin could keep alive a hybrid strain of mice that had developed fatal systemic lupus erythematosus, with only occasional reinforcement by pairing with cyclophosphamide. Thus, the placebo that produced an associative "learned" response, via the brain, had a therapeutic immunologic effect. (Amazingly, the 1926 work of Metal'nicov and Chorine of the Pasteur Institute had been overlooked. They were able to induce peritoneal inflammation by the mere warming or scratching of the skin after preliminary pairing with microbial extracts.) David and Suzanne Felten's mapping of sympathetic nervous system innervation of immune system organs (particularly the thymus) clarified that the immune system is "hardwired" to the brain in addition to its "softwiring" by circulating substances produced by the brain. Within immune organs, they showed that sympathetic nerves can end at junctions with lymphocytes in a way similar to junctions between nerves (synapses). Therefore, neurotransmitters produced by sympathetic nerve endings (norepinephrine and neuropeptide Y) can influence the development and function of immune cells; thus, the work of the Feltens furthered the integration of psychoneuroimmunology with neuroscience.

Gerard Renoux and colleagues carried psychoneuroimmunology to the cortex of the brain with the discovery of laterally differential effects on T cell maturation and function. Besedovsky and Sorkin demonstrated changes in corticosterone levels and firing rates of hypothalamic neurons after antigenic challenge, thus proving that the brain-endocrine-immune axis operates in *both* directions. The work of Korneva and Klimenko showing the spatial and temporal pattern of electrical activity in the hypothalamus following exposure to antigen provided further evidence of the immune system-to-brain aspect of psychoneuroimmunology. When they electrically stimulated these hypothalamic areas in synchrony with the natural antigen-induced firing, immunity was enhanced, but when the stimulation was out of sync, immune response was suppressed. As mentioned, in then doubted work, Blalock and Smith discovered that lymphocytes synthesize hormone ACTH and neuropeptide beta-endorphin. Their findings set the stage for the current flood of information about the effects of immune cytokines on the brain as well as the effects of brain-produced and—regulated substances (neurohormones, neurotransmitters, and neuropeptides) on immune cells.

Studies on human stress and immunity, first done in the context of space flight, have continued in naturalistic situations (such as bereavement, marital discord, examinations, and caretaking of patients with Alzheimer's disease) and laboratory settings (using experimental stressors such as mental arithmetic tasks). The effects of naturally occurring depressive illness on immunity have been particularly well-evaluated, first shown in regard to T cell function by Schleifer, Keller, and Stein and then in NK cell function by Irwin. Valuable experiments were begun by Laudenslager and Coe using primate models to understand better the effects of social stress. The milestone 1981 text, *Psychoneuroimmunology*, edited by Robert Ader, has 14 chapters. Bob had appropriately renamed the field by adding "neuro" in view of the role of the *brain* in psychosocial influences on immunity and in immunologic effects on behavior.

CHAPTER IV

DEFEATING THE ENEMIES OF IMMUNITY: HUMAN IMMUNODEFICIENCY VIRUS AND AGING

Sometimes, even by modifying the terrain,
I encourage the force of resistance
against the invading microbe.

Hippolyte Bernheim, 1891

People don't grow old.
When they stop growing, they become old.

Anonymous

The same year that Ader's text book *Psychoneuroimmunology* came out, UCLA Assistant Professor of Medicine, Michael Gottlieb (later to become a controversial figure and good friend) had been seeing gay patients with a constellation of unusual illnesses related to severe immune deficiency, particularly pneumonia caused by the usually resisted, ubiquitous microorganism *pneumocystis carinii* (PCP) and a form of cancer, Kaposi's sarcoma (KS), previously described only in elderly men of Mediterranean origin. Michael named the condition "Acquired Immune Deficiency Syndrome" or "AIDS" for short. Soon, it was also described in intravenous drug abusers and heterosexual persons from Haiti (where it is now thought to have been transmitted from African origins). An etiological agent had not yet been found. In 1984, Robert Gallo of the National Institutes of Health and Luc Montagnier of the Pasteur Institute in Paris discovered the agent—human immunodeficiency virus (HIV). At first, the virus was called human T cell lymphotropic virus III (HTLV III). HTLV I and II can cause leukemia. Both are retroviruses, as is HIV. A retrovirus is made of RNA, not DNA (the material of genes). The enzyme reverse transcriptase is responsible for converting an RNA virus into DNA material so that the virus can be incorporated into the genome of the cell that then replicates the virus. It was soon realized that HIV did not belong to the HTLV group of viruses. Now we know there are at least two HIVs. Both HIV-1 and HIV-2 are a cause of AIDS, the latter mainly in Africa. By 1985, a test for infection based upon the presence of antibody to HIV was developed. (Montagnier, whom I later first met at UCLA, probably had first discovered the virus, the subject of a patent, prestige, and ethics dispute between France and the United States.) In 1982, AIDS seemed to me to be an ideal disease to study from a psychoneuroimmunologic point of view. It was likely an infectious disease resisted by the immune system; it was definitely a disease of immune aberration (as were the autoimmune diseases that I had previously studied); it also appeared to involve the brain as manifested by AIDS dementia complex (ADC)—not surprising in that psychoneuroimmunology posits integral relationships and similarities between the brain and the immune system. Moreover, as will be more fully understood, I felt a personal, moral obligation to devote my professional talents to a better understanding of this horrible disease.

My eventual with my return to San Francisco coincided with the formation of the Biopsychosocial AIDS Project (BAP) at UCSF, headed by Lydia Temoshok, who is also known for her work on the "Type C" or cancer-prone personality. The goal of the project was to find psychological, immunologic, and health correlations in AIDS as well as to study psychosocial aspects of the incipient epidemic. I was warmly welcomed by its members, mostly psychologists. On the eve of conducting detailed surveys of personality, stress, psychological distress, social support, and, especially, sexual behavior, the issue arose as to whether or not all the interviewing psychologists (pre-or post-doctoral) should be gay. Lydia and I decided that the simplest way to determine whether the sexual orientation of the interviewer would bias the interview was to conduct a pilot test. In reviewing a series of videotaped interviews, neither Lydia nor I could discern differences in quality based on sexual orientation. (Of course, the straight interviewers could not have been homophobic; otherwise, they would not have volunteered for such a project.) We did some cross-sectional (one time only) studies comparing psychological factors with immunologic measures relevant to AIDS and ARC. [ARC, or AIDS-Related Complex, involves at least one AIDS-related symptom, but falls short of the criteria for AIDS established by the Centers for Disease Control (CDC).] We found, for example, that persons with AIDS who reported lower amounts of tension and anxiety had higher numbers of helper T cells, also known as CD4 or CD4+ cells. (HIV enters helper T cells and other cells through the CD4 receptor.) They also had higher levels of cytotoxic T cells (CD8 cells), natural killer (NK) cells, and a subset of CD8 cells felt to be virucidal. The single individual factor most highly statistically correlated with higher numbers of virucidal cells was the "ability to say 'no' to an unwanted favor". This assertiveness and ability to take care of oneself is the opposite of masochism, self-sacrifice, and emotional unexpressiveness that I (and others) had found common in persons with autoimmune disease or cancer. Our findings among persons with ARC, however, were not completely parallel to those of persons with AIDS, making clear the importance of longitudinal (repeat evaluation) studies.

A promising source of information on the development of AIDS was the newly formed, long-term Multicenter AIDS Cohort Study (MACS), a major public health study of HIV-infected gay men based in four cities: New York, San Francisco, Miami, and Los Angeles; however, the types of psychological information gathered from these cohorts was relatively meager. UCSF-BAP applied for a supplemental grant from the National Institute of Mental Health (NIMH) to do more extensive psychological analyses of the MACS participants at risk for AIDS. We planned to evaluate a group of approximately 1,000 gay men and a control group of 200 straight men living in the predominantly gay Castro district of San Francisco. Our collaborating immunologist would be Daniel Stites, head of clinical immunology at UCSF and co-author of a widely used medical textbook on the subject. (Dan had been a student in my psychiatric clerkship group at Stanford Medical School.) Dan is an able, generous, and open-minded immunologist in the genre of John Fahey at UCLA, both of whom are comfortable collaborating with behavioral scientists. The site visitors, scientists from various parts of the country evaluating the project for funding suitability on behalf of the NIMH, questioned our ability to get full cooperation for repeated questionnaire completion and blood testing from straight men. One of the gay psychologists responded eloquently that, because of the unique nature of San Francisco, he expected that straight men—particularly those from the Castro district—would share concerns about the epidemic, probably having friends afflicted by it. He said, "San Francisco is a community, not a city with a gay community, as you from other parts of the country may not realize." We got the money and, as expected, the cooperation of both gay and straight men at comparable rates of 93% and 85%, respectively.

I became interested in the exception to the rule—the long-survivor of AIDS. Why do some persons with AIDS live longer when treatment variables are equivalent? I maintained regular involvement with BAP in search of some of these answers, even after moving to Los Angeles, and it was this work that later interested writer and medical humanitarian, Norman Cousins. We informally studied a small group of individuals who had survived more than two years after their initial opportunistic infection or more than three years after development of Kaposi's sarcoma, since prognosis with the latter was then somewhat better than the former. These were the days prior to the availability of AZT (zidovidine), the first antiretroviral treatment for the disease (that works by inhibiting reverse transcriptase), and prior to the use of sulfa drugs (Bactrim® or Septra®) for prophylaxis of PCP. These rare individuals, 18 in all, seemed to possess a remarkable ability to adapt to and cope with life. From our pilot interviews (without a control group), we distilled a list of characteristics associated with long-survival:

1. Perceiving the treating physician as a collaborator and not interacting in a passive-complaint (or defiant) mode.
2. Having a sense of personal responsibility for one's health and a sense that one can influence health outcome.
3. Having a commitment to life in terms of "unfinished business", unmet goals, or as yet unfulfilled experiences and wishes.
4. Having a sense of meaningfulness and purpose in life.
5. Finding new meaning as a result of the illness itself.
6. A prior mastered experience with a life-threatening illness or very serious life event. (More of the long-survivors had this experience than could be expected but still not the majority.)
7. Engaging in physical fitness or exercise programs.
8. Deriving useful information from and supportive contact with a person with AIDS shortly following diagnosis.
9. Being altruistically involved with other AIDS patients.
10. Acceptance of the reality of the diagnosis of AIDS in conjunction with refusal to perceive the condition as a death sentence, or at least an imminent one.
11. A personalized means of active coping that is believed to have beneficial health effects.
12. An altered lifestyle to accommodate the disease in an adaptive manner.
13. Assertiveness and the ability to say "no".
14. The ability to withdraw from taxing involvements and to nurture oneself.
15. Sensitivity to one's body and one's psychosocial and physical needs.
16. An ability to communicate openly about concerns, including illness.

One of the things that stands out overall in the list is a sensitivity to one's own inner self—both physically and psychologically—and corresponding adaptive behavior; however, I learned that one cannot evaluate any particular characteristic of long-survivors without understanding its meaning to the individual. For example, the first time I came across a long-survivor who denied having an exercise regimen (after having produced our initial paper on long-survival), I suggested that he might wish to consider partaking of one, since it seemed to be helpful to others. By then, I also had had evidence that natural killer cell activity was enhanced by exercise in healthy old people. I explained, "I have come to think that perhaps the natural killer cell may be important in individuals whose helper T cells are low. Perhaps exercise is something you should think about to boost your NK activity."

"Absolutely not!"

"You seem to have strong feelings about that." (I *am* a psychiatrist, after all.)

"I certainly do. Prior to my becoming ill, I was a physical fitness nut. I went to the gym every day. I was extremely vain. I exercised while admiring myself in the mirror. I was concerned with my own beauty and being admired. I feel now that I was extraordinarily narcissistic and that I had a very shallow value system. Since I've gotten ill, I've totally changed my outlook and am very deeply concerned about others, which I feel is far more meaningful." He had found new meaning as a result of the illness. Thus, I have come to think that psychosocial research, particularly those involving questionnaires, is often superficial and potentially misleading.

One of the long-survivors that we studied was Michael Callen, who, at the time of his death in 1994, was the longest known survivor with symptomatic AIDS after 12 years of illness, which he battled heroically. Michael's first book, *Surviving AIDS*, told of our work at BAP. Michael epitomized every aspect of long-survivorship. He had lived life in the fast lane prior to falling ill, after which time he changed his lifestyle and had an enormously positive impact on the AIDS epidemic. (Later, we were to realize that these "turn-around" life experiences were important in a number of long-survivors.) Michael helped establish AIDS Projects San Francisco, New York, and Los Angeles that are designed to help AIDS patients find psychological and financial support; he lobbied Congress for AIDS research funding; his books provided hope to persons with AIDS. Michael's parents were present at his memorial service, having flown in from a rural town of 5,000 in agricultural Iowa. His brother, who sat with his arm around Michael's bereaved partner, spoke movingly about how Michael's example of concern and love for others had benefited his own marriage. There were a number of lesbians present at the service because of Michael's wish for unity between male and female homosexuals. As the lone survivor of Michael's quartet, a woman heart-wrenchingly sang a beautiful song that he had written. The ability to show humor through tears seemed to run in the family. Michael's brother comically told of taking Michael's ashes, held between his legs on the airplane, in order to be buried under the apple tree that they had planted together in their Iowa garden as children. Michael had instructed him to bury his ashes there because, after all, he himself was a "fruit" (gay man), and apples made good "tarts" (feminine gay men). People from all walks of life intermingled.

Susan and I became very good friends with another long-survivor, Bob Buchser. On sick leave from his job as a college professor, Bob decided to accomplish, before death, the restoration of a magnificent pair of large Victorian flats in a run-down neighborhood, of which he was the first to begin gentrification. The area, close to San Francisco's Opera House, has since become a beautiful district of shops, restaurants, and restorations. As his mother had died when he was quite young, Bob had been reared by his father who was now well into his 80s. Although he had been close to his father as a child, they had not been as close in adult years because his father had remarried and moved to a nearby city. Bob hired workmen but did most of the work himself; however, his father came to work with him day after day, returning home on weekends. When the magnificent building was fully restored, I worried that Bob would become ill—having met his goal. To the contrary, Bob chirped, "Well, since this turned out so well, I guess I'll buy another one to restore," which is exactly what he did.

I continued to see Bob when I would come up from Los Angeles to San Francisco. On one such occasion, Bob was quite ill, saying that he had been feeling terrible for a few days. His abdomen was swollen. I asked if I could feel his belly and palpated his liver, finding it grossly enlarged and extending almost into the pelvis. I suspected, and it was confirmed, that he had non-Hodgkin's lymphoma. His physician told me that he thought Bob had about three weeks to live, but would try treating him with chemotherapy. Bob recovered from lymphoma, of which there was no sign at autopsy two and a half years later. Rather than sitting around waiting to die, Bob chose to return to college teaching. What seemed to trigger Bob's death was the death of his father, to whom he had once again become so close. Since developing AIDS several years earlier, Bob had recovered not only from lymphoma but also three bouts of PCP, cryptococcus, and avian tuberculosis (MAI). Being an active seeker of new information and approaches, he had taken AZT as well as a variety of nonstandard therapies (including dextran sulfate and the Salk polio vaccine). He had been an advocate for those suffering from AIDS; he had had a fierce determination to live and an excellent support system of devoted friends. These remarkable long-survivor cases demonstrate that CD4 T cell numbers are by no means the whole story. Important clues toward conquering AIDS can be found in such individuals, who inevitably appear to be exceptional human beings as well as exceptional "cases".

Gail Ironson, M.D., Ph.D. (psychiatrist and psychologist), of the University of Miami, and I have synopsized the psychological characteristics described in studies of long-survivors into three general categories: positive expectancies; deep, meaningful life goals; and emotional expressiveness. Gail was interested in alternative therapies that many of our long-survivors reported using, such as massage. With the help of a large number of volunteer masseurs and masseuses, Gail had found that 45-minute massages four times a week for three months produced clinical improvement and CD4 T cell increases in patients with AIDS. She demonstrated the importance of touch, a neglected element in our contemporary hands-off style of medicine and our cultural tendency to perceive touch as sexual. The massage therapists had been rotated so that immune and health changes in the patient could be more clearly linked to touch and not to the development of a relationship with the therapist.

Subsequently, at UCLA, I undertook a psychoneuroimmunologic study of HIV positive persons who have very low levels of CD4 T cells (below 50/mm³ of blood) yet who remain asymptomatic for prolonged periods of time (at least more than nine months). Most of our original observations have held true with these persons as well. With immunologist John Fahey, I found a possible mediating mechanism: the presence of normal levels of natural killer (NK) cell activity. NK cells are nonspecific killers of virus-infected and cancer cells. NK cell cytoxicity usually starts to fall early in HIV infection and generally is very low by the time CD4 T cells are below 50. Since NK cells are nonspecific, they are not affected by the ability of the virus to mutate rapidly, which overwhelms the T cells. Perhaps the NK cell serves a backup function like those skinny, little spare tires in many new cars. They keep you going, albeit not as fast and not as far. Yet what keeps the NK activity up? NK cell cytoxicity (ability to kill cancer or virus-infected cells) is stimulated by a cytokine product of ever-diminishing CD4 T cells, interleukin-2 (IL-2) that has been tried therapeutically in AIDS. Interferon, like IL-2 a product of the "T helper 1" component of CD4 cells that is especially reduced as HIV infection progresses as well as by also-infected macrophages, stimulates NK cells and has been tried therapeutically. (It is helpful in Kaposi's sarcoma.) Low levels of IL-2 and interferon may account for the low levels of NK cytotoxicity in HIV/AIDS. However, the neuropeptide beta-endorphin, a product of the brain, may also promote NK cell activity. Beta-endorphin, an opioid which shares receptor sites with opiates like morphine, may be partially responsible for the sensation of pleasurable experience. The neuropeptide beta-endorphin, a product of the brain, is related (like the opiates such as morphine that it shares receptor sites with) may be involved in pleasurable experience. We have shown that it is responsible for the increase in NK activity induced by exercise. These are intriguing leads. In science, every new answer generates more questions.

Gail Ironson and I felt justified in applying for a large grant to study long-survival, not only in a one-time cross-sectional way but also in a prospective predictive design. We felt that two sites (Miami and Los Angeles) would be necessary to recruit a sufficient number of rare long-survivors falling into two groups: those having had AIDS (as defined by symptoms, not just CD4 cell count) for more than four years and those with no symptoms despite very low CD4 cell counts for a prolonged period of time (more than nine months). We then wanted to take asymptomatic persons at low, but not very low, CD4 counts (150-400) and follow them for three years with psychological and immunologic tests every 6 months using criteria developed for the study of long-survivors to predict who would get sick and die and who would continue to live on healthily. It was not funded. As will be discussed, this approach was seen as odd. We rewrote the proposal. It was turned down again. More than two years later, after the clinical situation for people with AIDS had been drastically altered for the better by the advent of protease inhibitor drugs, it was suddenly funded to the tune of $1.6 million ($200,000 less than requested for the five years). Obviously, NIH had some extra money at the end of the fiscal year that it did not want to return to the Treasury. Our long-survivor definition had to be modified to having been the case *prior* to taking the new drugs.

As our big NIH study got underway, we particularly sought a broad spectrum of persons with AIDS, people of low socioeconomic status, minorities, heterosexuals, women. Most AIDS research had been done on middle-class gay men. We decided to asses how the research subject deals with close-to-real-life situations. For example, we do a role play with a professional actor portraying an abrupt, rushed, impolite HMO physician who refuses to do an additional non-authorized viral load test (a newer, more accurate way of assessing disease status than CD4 cell count) after placing the patient on new medication he/she does not believe is helpful. Most longer survivors give that awful doctor hell—or change doctors!

There have been many fascinating hours spent with such remarkable people—some poignant, some tragic, some funny. The kind of fighting spirit that we have continued to see in our new research on long-survivors was charmingly illustrated in a young man from Texas who came to see me before the grant was obtained, having read about my interests. His CD4 T cell count was $10/mm^3$. (There are many thousands of cubic millimeters in the approximately 3 quarts of blood in the body.) About a year later, he called me from New York to let me know that he had moved because he wanted to stay in touch. I asked him, "How are your T cells?" "Well, I have only one, but I am so proud of him. He is the most powerful T cell in the whole world. He is the greatest." His tone changed, "I am beginning to think that's a bad attitude. If I lose him and go down to zero, I'm going to grieve, and work has shown that grief in HIV positive people is not good for their health." Instantly, he bounced back, "I changed my mind. I decided if he goes, I'll not be depressed at all because I'll write a paper that says T cells have nothing to do with AIDS." A health professional continuing to work full-time after having AIDS for six years told me, "A little psychosis helps." He had always considered himself a special person. After he got AIDS, he became convinced that he was the new "American Messiah". He had a direct connection to God, who would speak to him via the clouds. In response to the standard question, "To what do you attribute doing so well in the face of AIDS?", he replied, "How can you be so stupid after I've been talking frankly to you for almost an hour? Do you think Dad would let me down?" A lovely lady had been diagnosed with what was then referred to as GRID (gay-related immune deficiency) in 1980 after her bisexual husband had been diagnosed with the same condition. She developed full-blown AIDS in 1983 with wasting syndrome, her weight having dropped from 150 to 85. And she was still going strong in 1997! She was determined to live to care for her soon-to-be-born grandchild. One of her 15-year-old identical twin daughters had AIDS, zero CD4 cells, was refusing any medication, and was seven months pregnant. (Without medication and in the likely presence of a high maternal viral load, the baby would probably be born infected, as Mrs. Johnson well realized.) Interestingly, the also-HIV-infected twin was doing very well with 500 CD4 cells. She was in school and took good care of herself. The sick twin had run away from home and become a prostitute. Mrs. Johnson had lost to AIDS her husband, a counselor to whom she was close, and her best woman friend. She was engaged to be married to another bisexual man with AIDS and was prepared to care for him, too, if necessary.

Dr. Agnes Lin
441 N. Oakhurst Dr. Suite 604
Beverly Hills, CA 90210

It is now ironic to realize that long before the approach gained popularity, Lydia Temoshok and I wrote a paper in 1987 on the usefulness of a psychoneuroimmunologic perspective in AIDS research, namely on tying psychologic factors to immunologic ones. We had previously tried to organize a national conference on the topic but were unable to get funding from the NIMH. The idea seemed too "far out", just as my stress research on rats had seemed many years before. Fortunately, private resources came to the rescue, that time in the form of the Institute for the Advancement of Health, founded by Eileen Rockefeller Growald. Through her support, a small but worthwhile conference was held at a lovely site in rural New York, attended by all *eight* researchers in the world then interested in such an approach. Since that time, the NIMH has sponsored two major conferences on psychoneuroimmunology and HIV/AIDS. Obviously, by then the attendance was greater, since government funding agencies never fund anything that is not close to mainstream. Eventually, nearly all psychoneuroimmunology projects in *whatever area* (basic science, stress, etc.) became funded through the NIMH from monies allocated for AIDS research, a policy that ultimately proved to be politically unwise (and, I feel, ethically questionable, even though very useful and productive). I maintain that all institutes should be involved in supporting those aspects of psychoneuroimmunologic research relevant to their particular missions. Some AIDS activists became concerned that monies were being diverted from AIDS research to aspects of psychoneuroimmunology that were not AIDS-relevant. Thus, the decision to use relatively "easy money" for psychoneuroimmunology ultimately threatened the entire support of the field. Fortunately, *POZ Magazine*, aimed at the HIV-infected, as well as the controversial AIDS activist group ACT UP, supported PNI. Despite its subsequent precarious funding status, psychoneuroimmunology was chosen as the theme of the 1994 conference marking the reuniting of the National Institute of Mental Health with the National Institutes of Health (which I had felt should never have been separated in the first place, 34 years previously). Conference chairperson, Susan Blumenthal, M.D., head of women's health for the NIH, had selected psychoneuroimmunology as it represented a bridge between behavioral and biomedical sciences. I had the honor of giving the introductory lecture on the history of the field as well as the closing remarks, in which I made the recommendation (ignored, of course) that each institute designate a small proportion of its budget for psychoneuroimmunologic research relevant to the area of its mission.

A wonderful side benefit of my association with BAP at UCSF was the development of a longstanding friendship with Jeffrey Moulton, Ph.D., whose doctoral dissertation based on work with BAP had to do with the clinical course of AIDS and the patient's attribution of disease. Jeff found that those who were self-blaming ("Oh, if I just weren't gay", "Oh, if I just hadn't gone to the baths") did worse than those who attributed their illness to bad luck or chance. He also found that "internalized homophobia" (psychiatrically speaking, "ego dystonic homosexuality"), in which the person was not self-accepting, seemed to have bad prognostic implications. While at BAP, I also had the pleasure of collaborating with a separate group at UCSF headed by Thomas Coates whose outstanding and well-known work remains primarily concerned with behavior change that leads to prevention of infection. Tom and others, such as my friends and colleagues psychiatrist Steven Schleifer and immunologist Steven Keller, working in inner city Newark, have shown that knowledge about HIV/AIDS is not enough. A change of group cultural attitude is necessary for individual behavioral change.

One of the joys of my days at BAP was coauthoring, with another good friend, Christopher Mead, a paper on "Human and Psychosocial Considerations in the Treatment of the Gay Patient with AIDS or ARC", published in the *Journal of Humane Medicine* and selected as the offbeat journal's best paper of the year. (At that time, 70% of patients with AIDS were gay or bisexual.) The particular needs of the gay person with AIDS underscore the critical nature of the patient-physician relationship for *all* persons. For some patients, a diagnosis of AIDS/ARC means not only facing fear of having a little-understood, life-threatening disease but also experiencing the added distress of "coming out" as a gay man. As Jeffrey Moulton showed, those who tend to blame themselves for their illness or adopt the common societal view that illness is punishment for being gay have even higher levels of emotional distress. Later work at UCLA documented that distress is likely to have adverse medical consequences. A gay patient is also likely to be hypersensitive to the *physician's* attitudes, which may be seen as representative of society's. If a patient fails to perceive that the doctor is in reality not homophobic, then the physician may need to spell out his or her attitudes. Moreover, the physician may develop defensive armor to protect against feelings of impotence in dealing with the disease and to buffer the pain of watching so many young people die. Such apparent coldness and indifference is devastating to an effective patient-physician relationship. As we found with the long-survivors, a sense of control strongly lessens dysphoria and may lessen immunosuppression. Through offering alternatives to promote active coping with illness, the physician can enhance the patient's sense of control, a key characteristic of long-survivors. From a sense of control comes hope, which maintains one's motivation to take active steps to enhance health, to comply with medical treatment, to strengthen one's support system, to live longer. In the words of Norman Cousins, "I have seen too many cases when death predictions were delivered from high professional stations only to be gloriously refuted by patients for reasons having less to do with tangible biology than with the human spirit, admittedly a vague term but one that may well be the greatest force of all within the human arsenal." AIDS-related brain dysfunction, accompanied by lassitude, lack of motivation, and psychomotor retardation, may be confused with depression and consequent lack of compliance with treatment. Unfortunately, these symptoms may also be exacerbated by some AIDS treatments, particularly immunomodulatory cytokines such as interleukin-2 and interferon, a natural result of which is to induce feeling sick. Complicating matters even further, depression is frequently associated with chronic Epstein-Barr and other herpes group virus infections, which are ubiquitous in AIDS.

Standard demographic questionnaires and psychological tests are too nonspecific to measure adequately AIDS-related attitudes, emotions, and behaviors among nonheterosexual persons; therefore, we developed some of our own measurement instruments at BAP. Drafts of proposed instruments for "gay and bisexual" men with AIDS and ARC (before the development of testing for HIV antibody) were circulated to all members of BAP prior to the weekly, half-day general meeting. With some prior thought but with no definitive plan as to how to handle the issue, I said, "These questionnaires seem pretty appropriate for the gay population, but very few items are specifically relevant to bisexual men. Bisexual men with committed relationships generally have women partners, and their sexual activities may be more casual, even furtive, with actually greater risk of infection and obvious danger to the heterosexual community. Moreover, there is not a 'bisexual community' in the sense that there is a gay community in San Francisco, which meets important needs for social support, self-acceptance, and so forth. Bisexual people may feel quite isolated, accepted neither by straight nor gay worlds. Believe me; I know whereof I speak. Do you want to study gay men exclusively, or do you want to rework the instruments to make them also appropriate for bisexuals? If the latter, I'd be glad to help." The at-ease, but startled, group chose the latter. The instruments wound up much improved and more broadly relevant. The working atmosphere at BAP became even more close. I had surprised myself. While having confided in very few straight colleagues who were good friends, including Lydia, never had I "come out" professionally. I was both proud of myself and grateful for the BAP environment that enabled me to do so. I vowed never again to dissimulate, but neither would I advertise, since the issue is—or at least should be—professionally irrelevant.

I had hoped to remain at the main UCSF campus in San Francisco, continuing AIDS research with the congenial BAP group; however, the temporarily leaderless Department of Psychiatry was not in a position to provide funding or laboratory space. Chronic political infighting had led (and still leads in many universities) to the almost routine replacement of psychiatry department chairpersons. Since it was no longer possible to pursue PNI research at UCSF, I turned to my old friend Jolly West, who previously had offered me four different jobs affiliated with UCLA. [L. Jolyon West was Professor and Chair of UCLA's Department of Psychiatry and Biobehavioral Sciences. We had met originally at Stanford on the day of President Kennedy's assassination, a bonding experience.] Having had my fill of administration and psychopolitics in Fresno, I wished primarily to spend my time doing research and teaching. Jolly asked me what I would like to do. I replied, "You mean, what I *really* would like?"

"You may as well tell me."

"To do whatever work I wish, wherever I wish, both in Los Angeles and in San Francisco."

Jolly promptly found me the near-ideal position at one of the two UCLA-affiliated Veterans Affairs (VA) Medical Centers, an attractive four-square-block complex in the San Fernando Valley (Sepulveda), north of the university. I would have most of my time for research and teaching but would also have some clinical and administrative responsibilities as head of the Drug Dependency Treatment Unit.

At UCLA/Sepulveda VA Medical Center, I had planned to return to work on immunologic abnormalities, particularly autoimmunity, in mental illness—a subject that still remains murky. Schizophrenics have a propensity to form all sorts of autoantibodies. An autoimmune hypothesis of schizophrenia, as Jeffrey Fessel and I had postulated so long ago, remained attractive since schizophrenia and autoimmune diseases share the presence of autoantibodies, genetic and personality predispositions, and, at least sometimes, stress-induced precipitation. The pursuit of this line of research seemed practical since there were plenty of psychiatric patients at the VA, and I was being supplied with an immunologic laboratory and a "free" salaried immunologist. Although a nice person, the immunologist who was provided for me turned out to be, if not mentally ill himself, eccentric and impossible to work with. Understandably, I began to question the generosity of the offer; another nonfunctional VA employee was just being bumped to a different job. Thankfully, the immunologist had the prudence to leave the position and become a sculptor, an occupation for which he was far better suited. Along with him went my plans for again studying immune abnormalities in mental illness.

By a stroke of luck, right to Sepulveda came from South Africa, one of the most outstanding gerontologists in the world, endocrinologist John Morley. Although John had been a terrible undergraduate student, in rebellion against his parents who had pressured him to get an education rather than becoming a tennis pro, he eventually wound up being a Type A+++ personality, producing prodigious amounts of work. When I commented to John that his driven nature combined with no exercise and obesity was a set-up for a heart attack, his reply was, "So what? I already have more than 200 articles in top peer-reviewed journals." Given my interest in the exceptional individual, I approached John about studying very healthy elderly persons in the hope of determining whether life stress, failure of coping, and consequent emotional distress anteceded changes in immune function, which, in turn, anteceded illness and death. Although more scientifically valid, prospective studies are not often done because of their expense and difficulty. True to form, however, the challenge of a prospective study on healthy elders appealed to John.

Incidentally, John Morley, the former casual student turned super-scientist, is not the most extreme version of that subspecies, who have done much to advance knowledge at some price to their own all-roundedness. A visiting professor, whose work with one animal experimental model is meticulous and elegant, once remarked to me during dinner, "I work seven days a week, 10 hours a day."

"That must be hard on relationships."

"That's what all my wives have said."

"How many wives?"

"Five. But now I have a wonderful relationship with a molecular biologist. She works seven days week, 10 hours a day. You can't imagine how thrilling it is to awaken at 2 AM, roll over in bed, and begin talking about tumor necrosis factor alpha." This relationship will last.

To complete the "healthy old people" research team, I began hunting for a psychologist research assistant, nearly settling on an impressive young man who knew much of what I knew. Suddenly, it occurred to me that what I really needed was someone who knew what I *didn't* know. I then hit the jackpot in hiring geropsychologist Donna Benton, who had done postdoctoral training in geriatric psychology at the University of Southern California. Donna was a linchpin to the project in a number of ways—in her knowledge of geriatrics, in her congeniality which kept the elderly cohort intact, in her laid-back Type B personality which complemented my Type A-. Although Donna often pushed the limits of my patience *vis-à-vis* deadlines, tending to wait till the last minute to get something done, she never failed to come through. She and I remain good friends, and even though she is now on the faculty of the University of Southern California, she is helping me with the latest study of long-survivors with AIDS.

John, Donna, and I did a one-year study of immunologic and psychological parameters in 50 physically healthy people over the age of 65, the great majority being over 70. At the time of recruitment, these persons had no serious illness and were independently living. If they had ever been successfully treated for a serious illness, such as cancer, there had to have been no sign of recurrence for over five years. Most of the recruiting was done through senior centers at which they were active participants. As expected, the physically healthy elderly were found also to be remarkably psychologically healthy, with extremely good coping skills and no psychological distress (anxiety, depression, alienation). Somewhat surprisingly, they did not show signs of immunosenescence—age-related changes in immune function. The immunologic theory of aging proposes that genetically programmed immunosenescence is a prime determinant of maximum life span and is related to the onset of malignant, infectious, and autoimmune disorders with age. Different components of the immune system are not uniformly affected by aging. The most significant decrements occur in T cell immunity. In terms of humoral (antibody, B cell) immunity, the old person usually has difficulty in responding to new antigens but not to previously encountered ones (secondary or booster response). Thus, recall of old events remains intact but learning of new ones tends to become impaired in both old immunologic and nervous systems. Our elderly subjects, however, had immunologic functions equivalent to or better than those of our healthy 21 to 39-year-old control group. They also had the ability to remember recent as well as remote events (no signs of dementia). Both T cell (specific) and NK cell (nonspecific) functional abilities were unimpaired. Thus, both psychological well-being and immunologic intactness go together for a healthy old age. Many studies showing reduced immunity in the elderly may have been skewed because the subjects were residents of nursing homes rather than those leading vigorous, independent lives.

George Cochran was one of our healthy elderly people, who worked as a volunteer updating my reference files at least one day a week from the time he was 86 until he was nearly 94. George had been a successful industrial engineer. After retirement, he became active in various organizations, including being a regular volunteer at the VA, and he continued to lead a full and busy life. George faithfully went for an annual medical checkup. Nothing was ever wrong. We found that his immune system and mental capacity were indistinguishable from a young person's. He was totally alert with no defects in cognition. No depression. No anxiety. Just a delightful, charming, engaging, witty, humorous man. There was one thing that stymied him. "I can't understand why young people, including you," he gibed, "get hassled about trivia. What's the big deal?" George dated a charming younger (by one year) woman, one year younger than he.

One day, George invited me to lunch, suggesting, "Let's go in my car because I'm parked closer." As we approached the car, I asked, "What do you think of this car? My wife has one."

"I think it's a piece of junk."

"I do, too."

"I picked up copies of *Motor Trend* and *Car and Driver* and have been reading about the Cadillac Seville STS and its Northstar drive-train system. It seems that, finally, the Americans have come out with a really good car. I think I'll buy myself one because I need a car that'll hold up longer." Italian research on healthy centenarians (like ours) found them to be future-oriented.

When George suddenly developed optic neuritis, went blind, and could no longer be independent, I knew that he would soon die. He did. His funeral with a marvelous extended family was a celebration of life. George would really have enjoyed it.

Donna and I decided to ask the participants, who had initially agreed to be studied intensively on four different occasions over a period of a year, if they would be willing to be studied indefinitely on an annual basis. Thirty of our subjects committed to the longer study. Five years later, we were left with 23. Stubbornly refusing to cooperate with our research design, our participants did not develop serious illness, and only five died—three of sudden heart attacks. Thus, the number of deaths was too few for us to be able statistically to ascertain stress and immunologic antecedents of death. Although there is some six year follow-up data yet to be analyzed, we have already made some interesting observations. Both the immunologic and psychologic functions of the healthy elderly participants remained remarkably stable after five years. We created an unmarked lifeline representing birth to death, arbitrarily equivalent to 100 years. We would say to each person, "This line marks life. Put an X at the point of the line that reflects where you think you are in the course of life." My very funny, lighthearted, atypical Viennese postdoctoral student Peter Grohr analyzed these data. Those who estimated themselves to be older than their chronological age had lower levels of NK cell numbers and functioning than those who rated themselves as younger. The lifeline point, however, bore no relationship to illness. Is death a self-fulfilling prophecy? Can one can have an underlying awareness of impaired immunity?

Medical student Greg Hallert asked if he could do a research elective with me. Usually, I find that such short-term "help" is generally very time-consuming for me and not too productive for the student. I accepted Greg because he clearly was not the usual medical student. Having studied two years in Japan, he became an expert in martial arts (especially tai chi)—mental and spiritual components of which he finds most valuable. He is most interested in alternative or complementary modes of healing and their biological mechanisms. Obviously, Greg was a medical student for me. I set him up to analyze some of our data on psychological traits and immunity in our healthy elderly sample. He found that healthy old people with a strong need for control of events had higher levels of NK cell cytoxicity, as assessed on a per cell basis (the best way; one rarely reported) than those with less need for control. The findings in the comparison group of healthy young people was exactly the opposite. Thus, a personality characteristic that seems to be immunologically beneficial when old seems to be biologically disadvantageous when young. Such findings are, indeed, hard to interpret.

We decided to do some experimentation on our healthy elderly. Led by Maria Fiatarone of the Geriatric Research, Education, and Clinical Center at Sepulveda VA Medical Center, we used ergometric bicycles to assess the effects of aerobic exercise on immune function in young (control) and old persons. We would gradually build up the resistance until the participants quit from exhaustion. (We had difficulty getting Protection of Human Subjects Committee approval for this project because they were worried that the protocol might cause our elderly to drop dead.) The exercise resulted in increased NK cell numbers and function in both groups, but somewhat to our surprise, the average increase in NK cell activity was just as great or greater in the older as in the younger exercisers. (There was, however, greater variability in the amount of increase among the older subjects.) The increase lasted only about 10 minutes after exercise, roughly the same length of time it took to produce exhaustion.

To find out whether the increase in NK cell activity was mediated by the powerful NK cell stimulant, beta-endorphin (the endogenous opioid, or bodily-produced analgesic, responsible for "runner's high"), we repeated the exercise test in young women, first giving them a dose of naloxone, which blocks receptor sites for beta-endorphin and other endogenous opioids. Although the increase in numbers of circulating NK cells was not affected, each cell was less effective at killing target cancer cells. Killing is measured after treating *in vitro* target cells with radioactive chromium. When the cell is killed, the intracellular chromium is released into the surrounding supernatant fluid. The fluid is drawn off, and the amount of radioactivity in the supernatant is measured. Thus, exercise-induced increases in NK activity are opioid mediated, but increases in NK numbers are not. [Numerical increases are likely mediated by the catecholamines epinephrine and norepinephrine (adrenaline).]

One of my postdoctoral students was Hernan Rincón, now a consultation-liaison psychiatrist in Colombia, setting up PNI research there on allergy. Hernan, Donna, and I designed what we felt was an uncontroversial experiment to introduce, gentle, nonaerobic calisthenic exercise to frail, elderly men prone to falling. We would gradually build up to 45 minutes a day, three times a week, over a three-month period to try to induce lasting, not just transient, increases in immunity. To our dismay, we found a steady decline in the subjects' baseline NK cell activity and T cell responsiveness to mitogens. Moreover, transient increases in NK cell activity induced by exercise returned to baseline levels lower than what existed prior to exercise. Mild exercise appears to produce immune suppression in physically weak elderly persons, much like that which occurs in young athletes who are overtraining. Thus, one must introduce exercise with great caution and graduality in frail, elderly people.

Psychologist-psychophysiologist Bruce Naliboff (one of my all-time favorite coinvestigators) and I wondered whether mental stress would enhance immune function as physical stress (aerobics) had. Our healthy elderly participants were certainly as mentally sharp as their younger counterparts. We utilized a no-win mental stress task of subtracting the number seven from numbers in the thousands, while requesting that answers be given with every click of a metronome. Subjects were prompted to go faster and faster while being told of inaccuracies, the feedback being unrelated to actual performance. We found that the 10-minute mental stress task did, indeed, produce an acute rise in *numbers* of circulating NK and suppressor/cytotoxic T cells among young and old subjects, although increases in NK cell cytotoxic *activity* occurred only in young persons. Of the psychological reactions to the stressful task, only anger seemed to differ between the age groups, being greater in young subjects. We might speculate, therefore, that the absence of increased NK activity in the older group could have resulted from a difference in emotional reaction to the task. As a group, they found the task arousing but not as aversive as the younger subjects found it to be.

NK cell increases in physical and mental stress make teleological sense in that NK cells may not only serve as a backup for specific long-term immunity (as in preventing metastasis after primary tumor survival), but also they may serve as a first line nonspecific defense against virally-infected cells in emergency "fight or flight" situations. At such times, one would expect a defense mechanism that can attack microorganisms nonspecifically to compensate for the sacrificing of specific immunity for survival functions needed in the emergency. How long can a mammal flee a predator? To see how long this emergency-type mobilization of first-line defense goes on, Bruce developed a longer, no-win experimental stressor of an hour-long video game task that automatically becomes more difficult as a person's performance improves. Findings were similar to those of the 10-minute stressor.

Contrary to our expectations, we later found that in young men, pre-administration of the opiate antagonist, naloxone, did not block the mental stress-induced increase in NK cell activity, as it had in the case of exercise. Our curiosity about the relative contribution of emotional states to NK activity was further piqued by our discovery that the more emotional distress that a subject had experienced during the week before testing, the less his or her NK cell numbers increased during the mental arithmetic task. If the increase in NK cell numbers under brief stress is part of an adaptive response to potential injury, then our data suggest that chronic distress may impede normal immunologic adaptability.

There is clear evidence that naturally occurring life stress inhibitors various aspects of immune function in humans—the best work in this area being produced by Ronald Glaser and Janice Kiecolt-Glaser of Ohio State University. (An ideal husband-wife PNI research team, Ron is an immunologist and viral oncologist, and Jan is a clinical psychologist.) The Glasers have shown that both humoral and cellular immune defense mechanisms are compromised in medical students as a result of even *subacute stress* of examinations. (Examinations at

Ohio State University have historically been given during a single week and have been kept this way for the Glasers' research.) The students show how decrements not only in cellular (T and NK cell) immune functions but also in humoral (B cell) function, as demonstrated by a reduced ability to produce antibodies following immunization while under examination stress (the latter making the students at Ohio State just like my rats at Stanford!). Importantly, the Glasers have found increases in viral activation with these immune changes. Antibodies can serve as a marker of viral activity and replication for some viruses, such as herpes viruses. These viruses tend not be killed by antibodies that are produced in response to them. For example, Herpes simplex virus type 1 (the cause of cold sores or fever blisters) remains in the body after an initial infection in a latent, nonreplicating form and is kept in check by T cells; however, if T cell function is reduced, the virus replicates rapidly and triggers the production of more useless antibody. In this situation, the increase in antibody levels, usually indicative of a heightened immune response, is actually indicative of a weakened one. Besides laboratory evidence of compromised immunity during examination stress, there is an increased incidence of upper respiratory illness among medical students during that time. Furthermore, there are social (interpersonal) aspects of this immunosuppression, since the students who report being lonely during exam week fare the worst immunologically.

The Glasers and colleagues have also shown that the *chronic stress* of caregiving for a parent or spouse with Alzheimer's disease causes progressive declines in immune functions, more so as the condition of the patient deteriorates. Some recovery of immune function occurs when the patient begins receiving institutional care and the caretaker is relieved of much burden. Distress-related immunosuppression may have its most detrimental health consequences in older adult caregivers because of their often already compromised immune function. The Ohio State group also has shown that stress may enhance the propensity for cancer by way of a "triple threat": increased expression of genes promoting cancer (oncogenes, which are usually kept in check by suppressor genes), impaired ability of natural enzymes to repair defective DNA, and decreased immune surveillance and destruction of cancer cells. These findings have important implications for preventive medicine. My research underscores the importance of finding ways to *promote health*. It appears that the high rate of morbidity among older persons is not inevitable and that immunosenescence, which varies greatly, may be subject to "postponement". A better understanding of the psychoneuroimmunology of aging may make it possible for more persons to live long, healthy lives. It seems clear that both very healthy old persons and long-surviving HIV-infected individuals have good interpersonal and coping skills; they are not pessimistic or depressed; they lead meaningful lives. Thus, certain avenues of prevention seem apparent. People need social support, particularly during times of crises such as bereavement. They need to feel empowered to influence the course of their own lives and health. In this regard, group interventions may be useful. Depression should be recognized early and treated promptly because of its immunologic and health sequelae, which are particularly profound in the elderly and in those with immune-related diseases.

Exercise (inclusive of its psychological and social benefits) seems to have enhancing effects on immunity in young and old persons and, likely, in people with AIDS. Most of the long-surviving persons with AIDS who we studed had engaged in physical fitness programs and were sensitive to both their bodily and psychological needs. Such individuals "self-monitor" and exercise only to the degree that they feel capable. In persons with AIDS, we found that only fitness and regular exercise was significantly correlated with NK activity. These findings are compatible with research by Gail Ironson, Michael Antoni, Mary Ann Fletcher, and others of the University of Miami that demonstrated increases in helper T (CD4) cells in asymptomatic HIV-1 positive and negative gay males as a result of an aerobic exercise program. People should, likewise, pay attention to other good health habits like nutrition. Although the immune system is sensitive to protein deficiency, overeating and obesity likely impair immunity, since we know that moderate dietary restriction enhances longevity in rodents, as has been shown by Roy Walford of the UCLA Department of Pathology. Because the immune system is also sensitive to free radicals, a supplemental regimen of antioxidant vitamins and minerals, such as vitamins C and E, beta-carotene, minerals selenium and zinc, and the amino acid N-acetyl cysteine (NAC), may also be prudent—evidence for the latter being especially strong in HIV-infected persons.

It is of note that all of the very healthy elderly persons that we studied had incomes at least adequate to meet their basic needs. Obviously, people without means are likely to have poorer health habits, less access to preventive health care resources, and substandard nutrition. In addition, they bear the psychological stress of inadequate housing, no transportation, neighborhood crime, and so forth. All of these may serve as exponential risk factors for disease. It seems no wonder that low socioeconomic status is associated with higher morbidity and mortality. Psychoneuroimmunology has relevance to public health.

More prospective studies of late middle age and early old age are needed to determine how life stress, failure of coping, and dysphoria affect a variety of immune functions and whether these changes in immunity precede illness and death. Greater efforts also need to be made to determine whether coping skills training, stress management, social support groups, exercise programs, and other therapeutic approaches are immune enhancing as well as health enhancing. Donna Benton and I have made a grant proposal to investigate whether therapy to the enhancement of coping skills and self-nurturing in familial caregivers of Alzheimer's patients can prevent immunosuppression. Fawzy I. Fawzy, friend and psychiatrist colleague on the Psychoneuroimmunology Task Force at UCLA, found that a six-week psychoeducational program (consisting of medical education, relaxation training, problem solving, and group support) could facilitate improvements in psychological well-being, immunity, and of course of disease in patients surgically treated for malignant melanoma. (The group was co-led by Norman Cousins.) In a six-year follow-up, he found that program participants fared strikingly better in cancer recurrence and survival than patients who received only standard medical treatment; their mortality rates were lower than national and other institutional norms. Furthermore, Fawzy's data showed that life coping skills (whether in existence at the outset or developed over time) and initial tumor depth were the most important factors in predicting long range health. Consequently, the Department of Psychiatry has published an educational booklet written by Fawzy to be given to all cancer patients at UCLA Medical Center. Fawzy's study suggests that a low cost, simple-to-administer, short-term, psychoeducational program can have a significant long-term impact on health with concomitant savings in health care costs. Outcome studies of such programs should include economic impact, not only in terms of its direct medical costs but also in terms of work absenteeism, disability payments, and the like.

PART II

PSYCHOSOCIAL

CHAPTER V

WEIRDOES—PATIENTS AND OTHERWISE

To endure life is the primary duty of all living beings.
Illusion is of no value if it makes this more difficult.

Sigmund Freud

When I first came to Stanford, I was given the assignment of running one of three wards in the 96-bed Psychiatry Training and Research Section at the Palo Alto Veterans Administration Hospital. My first associate was Irvin Yalom, generally considered the world's authority on group psychotherapy, who in recent years has become known as a novelist utilizing psychological themes. Irv and I were a great team, despite the fact that Irv couldn't stand working on the inpatient unit. During this time, I became convinced that both psychodynamic factors and biology play a causal role in mental illness, as psychoneuroimmunology has since found to be the case in much of physical illness. Unfortunately, psychiatry now tends to have a purely biological orientation toward the etiology and management of mental illness. I believe that this skew, even worse than psychiatry's former strongly psychoanalytic bias, is a major factor in the decreasing choice of psychiatry for specialty training by medical students.

Russell was a patient in his early 30s who had suffered from paranoid schizophrenia for five years. His prognosis was technically good in that the break had occurred rather suddenly, while he had been under stress, and he had had a high level of functioning prior to his illness. Russell had worked in a sawmill in Northern California and had been married, with two children. Either he or his wife carried a very rare dominant autosomal (one gene) disease similar in its genetic transmittability to Huntington's disease. His first child inherited the disease and, though mentally normal, was born with deformed limbs. After the second child was born with the same disorder, Russell's schizophrenic break occurred.

During his five-year bout of schizophrenia, Russell had been given the antipsychotic drug Thorazine®. His sensitivity to the medication caused him to develop movement disorder side effects. Unfortunately, the maximum dose that he could tolerate was ineffective at controlling the schizophrenia, so Russell was given a long course of electroconvulsive therapy (much more effective for mood disorders, such as depression or manic depression). That failed, too.

I felt that there was one remaining way of helping this young man: individual psychotherapy. Such intensive work with mentally ill patients is virtually unheard of these days because the psychotherapeutic side of psychiatry is becoming somewhat of a lost art, particularly for the most difficult cases. Successful psychotherapeutic work with highly mentally ill patients has historically been accomplished by a gifted few.

While I could not place myself in the same league as these giants, I nonetheless decided to take this "incurable" case not only because of its difficulty but also out of compassion for the patient. Russell was paranoid, grandiose, and delusional—most of the time believing he was Jesus Christ. I saw him three times a week for the usual 50-minute hours, like the "old days" of psychiatry residency. I was getting nowhere with Russell. Although he would converse, it would only be about neutral subjects and not anything personal. When I tried to skirt his delusional system, he would only talk about the weather, current events, what was going on in the ward.

After many weeks of this, I commented, "You know, we seem unable to establish any relationship, and the treatment can only be effective if there is one."

"You are wrong. If I told you anything, you would broadcast my secrets to the world. I don't tell you anything; therefore, I don't hate you, and we get along fine." Later, the situation improved a little, "Maybe I'd tell you a thing or two, but the Communists have microphones hidden in the walls and are broadcasting everything I say to the world."

At the nine-month point of getting nowhere with Russell, the chronically ill patients from my ward (who had not responded to treatment) were being transferred to the "back wards" of the Menlo Park Division of the VA Hospital because my first research project on immunologic abnormalities in schizophrenia required the use of most of the beds. Patients who were well enough to function on an outpatient basis would be discharged. Russell was clearly one of the patients who had not gotten well. As a form of "shock" therapy, I informed him of the impending transfer, "Since these [Menlo Park Division] wards are not teaching units, they are poorly staffed. Though they are not horrible, they are not very pleasant—being full of chronically ill patients with relatively little programming. Why don't you take the shuttle bus, look at the ward, and see for yourself where you're going to have to be if you can't deal with things that are related to your illness?"

"I have no intention of going over there," he retorted. "Send me there if you want. I don't care where I live. It makes absolutely no difference to me whatsoever. After all, I'm Jesus Christ and I'm above all that. My environment is irrelevant."

At my last visit with him before his transfer, I sat across from him feeling most discouraged, and tears started rolling down my cheeks. Russell responded incredulously, abandoning his usual classic schizophrenic, "flat" affect, "You're crying!"

"Why not? You have now had every treatment known for mental illness—namely, medication, electroconvulsive therapy, and psychotherapy—and none of them have worked. You're going to be a chronic gorked-out patient likely for the rest of your life, and I think that's a tragedy. Moreover, frankly, I feel a great sense of personal failure. Perhaps grandiosely, I tried very, very hard to help, and clearly I have failed."

"You mean I've created a feeling in you; you feel something because of me? [Now don't forget, this was "Jesus Christ". Grandiose delusions often represent a defense against feelings of nothingness and unimportance.] My mother never felt anything. She kept the house clean; she kept me clean. She dusted me off like the furniture. Once at a Christmas party she ventured to take a drink and actually laughed. I cried because I thought she was sick. When I was in the hospital after breaking my leg playing high school football, she never came to see me." He announced, "Now I'm going to tell you something. My mother bathed me until I was fourteen. One day I got a hard-on while in the bath and screamed, 'Get out of here! Get out of here!'" Russell pleaded, "I couldn't help those feelings, could I? I have two daughters, and if they were teenagers, I'd never think of bathing them. She shouldn't have been bathing me, should she? I couldn't help it, could I?"

"Of course not. Her behavior was most inappropriate, and those feelings were elicited by that inappropriate behavior."

"I bet she had sexual feelings for me."

"I don't know what your mother's feelings were, but that certainly is a possibility."

"Doc, I believe I told you once that my father, whom I haven't seen in more than ten years and who had been an alcoholic but is now sober and long divorced from my mother, lives not far from here—in Salinas. Could I have a weekend pass and go visit my father?" (Russell had never asked for a pass before.)

"Of course you can."

When Russell came back from the visit, all delusions were gone and all symptoms of schizophrenia had disappeared. He reported, "I had a wonderful conversation with my father. He told me what a bitch my mother was." Russell was discharged within two weeks. He got his old job back at the sawmill in Northern California. I heard from him every year at Christmastime for a number of years. Russell's wife, understandably, had divorced him while he was in the hospital, but he would visit his children and occasionally date. He generally led a loner-type life, never remarrying but functioning. I heard from him for at least a decade following his discharge, during which time he neither relapsed nor required any further treatment or medication.

This kind of case raises several issues: Are the organic neurotransmitter abnormalities in schizophrenia the primary cause of the disorder or are they a by-product of another (for example, emotional or immunologic) process? Is there just a vulnerability to schizophrenia? Can biochemistry be changed by behavior just as behavior can be changed by biochemistry? Are the complex interactions of the organic and the psychological inextricably intertwined in mental illness—just as they are in physical illness?

Another case in point. A young Stanford assistant professor in the humanities, Joel, suffered a very acute psychotic break. He had taken a razor blade and slashed all over his accessible body—limbs, abdomen, chest, and so forth. Although they required a lot of sutures, none of the wounds was terribly deep or life threatening. At the time of hospitalization, Joel had the delusion that he was a pig. He refused to stand and would only move about on all fours, "oinking". Joel vehemently refused to bathe and was forcibly washed in the shower by attendants whenever his body odor became obvious. After some time on medication, Joel ceased to be a pig and requested psychotherapy. I worked with this brilliant young man in individual as well as group therapy. He had had a highly pathological, enmeshed, ambivalent relationship with his mother, of the sort once referred to as "schizophrenogenic". Joel improved to the point of stating that he was ready for discharge and would manage fine in the community if we could obtain a secure job for him at the VA as a janitor. Since this was a far cry from his status as a young Stanford professor, I recommended to him that he remain in treatment a while longer. (There was no limit to how long we could keep patients at the VA's expense at that time.)

Then a dramatic event occurred. Joel's father informed me by telephone that his middle-aged mother would be entering Stanford hospital for risky open heart surgery. The message was transmitted to Joel. A second call from his father reported that his mother had died on the operating table. It was now my burden to relay this news to

Joel, and I was afraid that he would regress from neat, clean aspiring janitor back to pig again. I told him.

Immediately, all symptoms disappeared. Joel became completely rational and apparently indistinguishable from his premorbid state. Everyone was amazed, myself included. In group therapy, he reflected, "I guess I had to get rid of her outside myself before I could get rid of her inside myself." Joel then announced his engagement to the chief nurse on the ward! We were all shocked, having been completely unaware of his intimacy with the nurse.

I encouraged Joel to rethink his relationship with the nurse, "What kind of person falls in love with someone as sick and regressed as you were? Does she love you because you're sick or in spite of the fact that you were sick because you have so many wonderful qualities as a human being that were pretty well masked during your illness?"

"This is the first time that I have ever felt truly loved," he replied unwaveringly. "If she could love me even when she had seen me as a pig, then she must truly care for me." Joel resigned his position at Stanford and took a comparable position at a university in another state. The nurse accompanied him. I heard from them periodically over the course of several years: happily married . . . couple of kids . . . no relapse. Although emotional and sexual involvement between health professionals and their patients is—and should be—condemned, perhaps the outcome isn't inevitably tragic.

One of the psychological theories of schizophrenia was the "double bind" theory, elaborated upon by the late Don Jackson and the late Gregory Bateson (once husband of Margaret Mead and an anthropologist who sought patterns and meaning in schizophrenic gibberish, later in dolphin communication). In the double bind theory, children who are continually given contradictory messages (verbally and/ or nonverbally) are more prone to developing schizophrenia in later years. The classic double bind, or "crazymaking", pattern involves a youngster's inability to comment on conflicting messages because the parent either denies having given them or criticizes the child for responding to what is always the "wrong" one of the mixed messages.

To illustrate this theory, I once observed in-house research at the National Institute of Mental Health headed by Lyman Wynn, who was experimenting with the use of new video recording technology in patient interviews. I watched one of the interviews through the one-way mirror, commonly used in psychiatric training. (From the side where the light is on, the mirror appears normal; what is going on can be seen from the other, unlit, side.) Lyman was doing a research interview with a father, mother, and son, a fairly silent and sullen young man of about 20. During a portion of the interview, the father (obviously a middle class government bureaucrat) said to the young man, "Son, I want to know whether you plan to go on to college or not because your illness has certainly interrupted your college plans and I have $20,000 [a lot of money at that time] that I've saved in an account that was to pay for your college education. Now, my brother who, as you know, is a big-time building contractor out West, is putting up a large development in Southern California and tells me that if I were able to invest that money in his project, I could triple it in two or three years. Being of modest means, I must make a decision about whether or not to invest the money that has been saved. There-fore, I want to know if I can have the money from your savings ac-count that we've saved for you."

"Keep your fuckin' money," the son retorted.

"Oh, son, I'm so disappointed that you're not interested in going to college," the father replied, obviously thrilled to be able to use the money.

The following situation illustrates the vital need for an appropri-ate array of treatments and settings for the chronically mentally ill, now so neglected. Psychopharmacologic management of mental ill-ness, a great advance, needs to be integrated with knowledge of the patient, appropriate use of custody, and provision of a supportive envi-ronment for those unable to function independently. (Surveys show that about one-third of the homeless wandering the streets are men-tally ill and one-third are drug addicted.)

I was requested by the UCSF attorney to consider offering expert testimony (in light of my later acquired background in forensic psychiatry) on behalf of the university, which was being sued in a medical malpractice civil suit. A young couple had a first child about six months old. One evening, just after the father had returned from work, the mother said, "We've run out of disposable diapers. I've been with the kid all day. You take care of her while I roller-skate over to the neighborhood store and buy some Pampers®. It will be a lot faster than your walking, anyway." She never returned. On her way home, her head was bludgeoned in with one of her roller skates.

The killer was soon apprehended. Since nearly all California state mental hospitals had been closed by then, he had been an outpatient at a clinic staffed by UCSF but funded by the City and County of San Francisco. I personally knew that the Director of the clinic was a competent young psychiatrist, since he had been Chief Resident in Psychiatry at Stanford when I was on the faculty there. Moreover, I had visited him while he was doing field work in rural Malaysia as a postresidency fellow in social psychiatry. The killer had been residing in a halfway house supervised by another competent member of the UCSF clinical faculty; however, supervision may have been somewhat lax at that particular time because the doctor's wife was in the hospital dying of cancer. Notes in the halfway house chart stated that the patient had been suffering from urethritis, and an appointment had been made for him at the UCSF Urology Clinic. The suit alleged negligence in that a patient that sick and clearly dangerous to be treated anywhere other than in a locked inpatient setting. The patient, Albert, had no prior history of violence but had been suffering from schizophrenia for many years.

At his trial for murder, Albert was adjudicated not guilty by reason of insanity because of his inability to know right from wrong as a result of severe mental illness. He was remanded to Atascadero State Hospital for the criminally insane. I went to Atascadero to examine Albert, who was by then in partial remission because of treatment with high doses of antipsychotic medication. I inquired, "What led you to kill that young lady?"

"I believed that in order to become an adult one had to perform the initiation rite of killing someone."

"What made you feel that you had to kill someone to become an adult?"

(With no emotion) "Why, everyone knows that adults get away with murder." (A classic example of "concrete" or literal schizophrenic "paralogic".)

"And how did you pick that particular victim?"

"Well, I had no weapon. She was tiny. Besides, she was wearing roller skates that I figured I could use to bash her head in with."

"Had you told your doctor at the clinic your idea [delusion] about having to kill to be an adult?"

"Of course not. He was an adult and would have killed me."

"Did you tell anyone at the halfway house?"

"No, they were adults, too."

"Were you taking your [antipsychotic] medication?"

"Yes, I was shoving the pills up my urethra." (I guess that absorption of medication through the gastrointestinal tract is better than through the urinary tract.)

Obviously, Albert was very mentally ill. The best treatment for him would have been in an inpatient facility, but the mental hospitals had been closed, overtly as part of "humane" deinstitutionalization. The covert reason (with which psychiatry naively colluded) was to reduce the state's mental health budget. [California ranked number two in the nation in *per capita* mental health spending under Governor Edmund ("Pat") Brown (1959-1966]. Under the governorships of his son, Jerry, and later Ronald Reagan, it dropped in ranking to 39th place.) Sue the state, not its university! How could the clinic doctor have known that Albert was imminently dangerous and, therefore, could be subject to (relatively brief) involuntary hospitalization? Thus, how could UCSF be liable? I felt that the case, although tragic, was defensible.

The university offered the devastated young husband and father an out-of-court settlement of $900,000. He refused. In the end, the university paid well over a million dollars.

The community mental health movement and deinstitutionalization of the mentally ill were based on two false premises. The first was that good psychiatric treatment would be effective for all mentally ill patients. Of course, good treatment is much more effective than bad treatment, but the best oncologists do not cure all cases of cancer. Likewise, a treatment team of the world's best psychopharmacologist working in collaboration with the world's greatest psychoanalyst could not cure every schizophrenic. The chronically mentally ill remain among us, and facilities for them are grossly inadequate. The second fallacy was that excellent community-based treatment with a broad range of services (including acute and longer-term inpatient units) is cheaper than hospitalization. Expensive community-based mental health became the natural target of government budget cutting. (Such is exactly what happened, as will be illustrated later.) By comparison, good community mental health programs are far more cost-effective than organ transplants!

Although most mentally ill people are not violent, and most violent persons are not mentally ill, we must face the fact that more mentally ill than sane individuals are violent. Increasingly more mentally ill persons are winding up in jails and prisons, in part because of "institution-seeking behavior" resulting from the inability to function in a nonstructured setting. A good survey funded by the California State Legislature, as a result of lobbying by the California Medical Association (when I chaired its Committee on Mental Health) and the California Psychiatric Association (when I served on its Council), found that about 20% of the inmates of five representative county jails had serious diagnosable psychiatric illnesses other than substance abuse. "Criminalization" of the mentally ill continues with high numbers of them kept in prisons, where treatment is abysmal and the psychiatrically disturbed are often abused by other prisoners.

One of the members of a psychotherapy group that I co-led with my father reported a fascinating recurrent dream that evoked some unusual interpretations by him which not only influenced my thinking but also had some impact on psychoanalysis itself. Xenia's dream went as follows:

"There is a giant lying on the grass. There is a big round circle above him indicating that he is dreaming, like in the comic strips. I'm in that dream just doing extraordinary things. I get the idea that I exist only in his dream. It is important for him to stay asleep because, if he wakes up, I will disappear. This is a tremendous fear."

Xenia was a 36-year-old single woman who entered analysis because of severe anxiety over recurring thoughts of becoming psychotic like her brother, who was a patient in a mental hospital. Her father, a physician, had urged her to get assistance for her extreme obesity. Xenia was neither seriously concerned about her weight, which probably exceeded 250 pounds, nor desirous of changing her eating habits. Fearful of men and marriage, she used her obesity to ward off romantic involvement. Although her homosexual inclinations were well defined, she showed no overt homosexual behavior. Xenia knew many people, but never allowed herself to be close to anyone, male or female. She was, however, devoted to her two dogs. Being highly loquacious and speaking loudly, as if addressing a huge audience, she continually gave the impression that she must make her presence known; however, she considered herself insignificant, surprised when others recognized her or listened to what she had to say. Xenia thought of herself as a thoroughly dependent person, which she indeed was, but acted in a bossy, officiously managerial way whenever possible.

As a child, Xenia never wanted to be a girl. She played football with the boys, carefully avoiding girlish activities, and now possessed an exaggerated interest in spectator sports. From an early age, she centered her thinking around the idea that her very existence was contingent upon the maintenance of a masculine image (patterned largely after her father) which led her to eat like a man and talk like a man. An early memory of her father eating a poached egg on toast in four bites impressed her considerably. Xenia saw very little of her parents, both being busy physicians. Her mother, the more aggressive and authoritarian of the two, was responsible for the care—and punishment—of the children. Xenia functioned to her own satisfaction until age 25, when her mother died. Shortly thereafter, her maternal grandparents died, and her brother became psychotic. As she watched him develop delusions of being Jesus Christ, her fears of insanity took hold; her character traits and compulsive actions intensified.

Although Xenia professed a great deal of hostility toward and fear of her father, it was revealed in analysis that her greatest moments of gratification came from being at home while her father was asleep. Her loud talk and eating habits were related to dinnertime dynamics when her father was home. Therefore, the recurrent dream represented Xenia's enjoyment of her father's presence at home, the absence of his criticism when he was asleep, and his tendency to leave or ignore her when he was awake. The groundwork for her underlying fears of abandonment and oral preoccupations had been laid earlier when her mother, because of illness, left her for a period of nine months beginning when she was one and a half years old.

Whether by accident or by unconscious motivation set in motion by Xenia's dream, Dad picked up Lewis Carroll's *Through the Looking Glass* and spotted the following passage about the sleeping Red King (King of Hearts):

He's dreaming now," said Tweedledee, "and what do you think he's dreaming about?"

Alice said, "Nobody can guess that."

"Why, about *you*!" Tweedledee exclaimed, clapping his hands triumphantly. "And if he left off dreaming about you, where do you suppose you'd be?"

"Where I am now, of course," said Alice.

"Not you!" Tweedledee retorted contemptuously, "You'd be nowhere. Why, you're only a sort of thing in his dream!"

"If that there King was to wake," added Tweedledum, "you'd go out—bang!—just like a candle!"

"I shouldn't!" Alice exclaimed indignantly.

For a long time, Xenia steadfastly denied ever having read or heard anything of *Alice in Wonderland* or *Through the Looking Glass*. Later, she admitted that she may have glanced at them, but never liked them. If she *had* heard the story of the Red King, she probably repressed it because of her need to deny her emotional needs for her father. We felt that it was likely, however, that Xenia's dream arose from purely intrinsic sources and conjectured that Lewis Carroll's fertile imagination and Xenia's neurotic imagery must have originated from comparable sources.

Dad was masterful at integrative thinking and deriving meaning from metaphor. He figured out that Xenia's basic "need for attention", such a universal motivation in childhood, was actually a search for reassurance that her image would appear in the mind of an important person in her life, her father. The anxiety experienced by Xenia can well be described as "existential anxiety". Xenia was worried that if her image were not present in her father's mind, she would no longer exist. This fear led Dad to redefine the basic human anxiety which, according to psychoanalytic theory, is fear of castration. Dad felt that it was not fear of castration but *fear of nonbeing*. In other words, before you can figure out *who* you are—the basis for adolescent identity formation, as described by Erik Erikson—you must know *that* you are. "I am" has to precede "who I am". Dad said that Descartes' "cogito ergo sum" (I think; therefore, I am) might better be stated in the passive voice "Cogitor ergo sum" (I am thought about; therefore I am).

From Dad's point of view, the process of therapy should not be limited to removing conflicts like castration anxiety, but should involve adding something to complete one's sense of self. He believed that therapy requires *synthesis*, not only analysis. Correspondingly, Xenia was able to relinquish her survival defenses, which were pointed out in individual therapy, only after she had established a state of existence in the individual and group therapeutic situations. Insights enabled Xenia to pull her life together. Years later, she spotted me at the San Francisco Opera House where she, about 100 pounds lighter, introduced me to her lesbian partner.

Dad's theory that the need for attention stems from a sense of nonbeing was dramatically displayed in a patient who worked with me individually. The patient, Wilkes, was a dashing, young assistant professor at Stanford whose specialty was the history of furniture. (Yes, furniture.) Wilkes got *his* attention by charm and charisma. He was the life of the party, a spellbinding raconteur, a teacher so captivating that his classes were always oversubscribed. Although married, he regularly tried to seduce both women and men. If he could not amuse, instruct, charm, entertain, or seduce, he would launch a verbal attack to ensure at least an angry reaction—better than none at all.

It turned out that Wilkes's parents had been abusive alcoholics.

As a child, when they were drunk and fighting, he would hide under the heavy Victorian dining table and cling in terror to its large center pedestal—the only place he felt safe. His love object was the antique table. The work with Xenia helped me greatly to understand Wilkes's need to be noticed and his ability to love only an inanimate object. These insights freed him to relate to others in a genuine, trusting manner without having to elicit reactions from them. Wilkes eventually remarried successfully.

As both clinician and researcher, I was not only influenced by my father, but also by the San Francisco Bay Area counterculture climate of the '60s. Commonly referred to as the "hippie age", the '60s fostered new ways of looking at accepted conventions; for example, the experiential movement in psychology was an outgrowth of this period. As encounter groups were the rage at the time, there was pressure on the psychiatry faculty from the medical students to provide some experiential training. I agreed to conduct a weekend encounter for a volunteer group of medical students on the condition that it would be utilized for the purpose of personal growth and not for conflict resolution. Significantly troubled individuals would be screened out by the medical students themselves. I also stipulated that I have a private room in which to sleep, although I, too, would be bringing a sleeping bag. The function was to be student arranged; I was merely to be the facilitator (not therapist).

On the weekend of the event, I was picked up by a psychedelically painted Volkswagen hippie van jammed with people, the driver of which was not a medical student. The driver, who was to be included in the weekend experience, was a groupie of author Ken Kesey, one of his "merry pranksters" from the La Honda area behind Stanford. The encounter was held at a nice home with a lovely view in the hills near La Honda. The first order of business, I felt, was to establish some ground rules for the weekend—confidentiality being a major item. As I began, this nonstudent chap began leaping back and forth across the furniture like a kangaroo. What ensued was a battle for control between him and me. After about a half an hour of this struggle, during which time I became increasingly annoyed, he disappeared into the kitchen. Moments later, he reappeared behind me in a surprise attack of peanut butter and mayonnaise, which he smeared all over my face and head while repudiatingly chiding, "It is difficult to be as pompous as you are when you look as ridiculous as you do." Everyone was hysterical with laughter. I gave up and proposed the following deal: I would put in abeyance my usual interpretive psychiatric commentary on group process in favor of experiential participation if the disruptive young man would, conversely, try to look at things analytically—not with his right "experiential" brain but with his left "rational" brain (whatever of it was still functioning). I remarked that we both might get something out of the experience. The group went extremely well and, with his intuitiveness, the brazen oddball turned out to be its most valuable member. When evening came, the group decided to create a communal sleeping arrangement by laying open sleeping bags all over the floor with a second layer of bags on top, rather than having each person sleep in his or her own bag Obviously no longer able to follow my initial plan of sleeping alone, I anxiously flopped down first so that I would not have to choose the person next to whom I would sleep. Wouldn't you know it? The first one to settle next to me was the driver. Then a pretty female student lay down on the other side. It was a bit uncomfortable as they held hands across my belly, but I "went with the flow".

My introduction to the '60s encounter group phenomenon was greatly enhanced by having been a classmate of Michael Murphy, the founder (with the late Richard Price) of the Esalen Institute in Big Sur, California, which was a haven for those seeking alternative mind and body therapies. Although he had initially started out as a premed, Michael was deeply influenced by the study of comparative religions and, following college, spent almost a decade in Asia as a Zen Buddhist monk. Esalen was an oasis for the likes of Gestalt therapy founder Fritz Perls, charismatic group therapist Will Schutz, and peculiar LSD therapist Stanislaus Grof, M.D., who specializes in hyperventilation therapy, now that LSD is illegal.

At Esalen, I became interested in alternative healing techniques, particularly bodywork therapies such as Rolfing, Feldenkrais, and the

Alexander technique. [Their founders (like Ida Rolf whom I knew) were gifted, but tended to make no scientific sense whatsoever in trying to "explain" their often effective work. Later, I tried to understand biological mechanisms underlying the efficacy of alternative and traditional healing methods in the context of psychoneuroimmunology.] I believe that body-based therapies give people more inner somatic awareness. It seems to me that somatic awareness (as psychoneuroimmunology has revealed, partially based on messages from immune system to brain) bears a similar relationship to physical health as psychological insight does to mental health.

My ties with Esalen are still strong. For a number of years, Margaret Kemeny, Ph.D., of UCLA, and I jointly gave an annual course in psychoneuroimmunology at Esalen, which is much more subdued than it was in its encounter group days. Also, I have teamed up with a gifted movement therapist and professional dancer, Jamie McHugh, to give a unique seminar at Esalen from both experiential and scientific frames of reference.

This more radical phase of my life led me to believe in experiential training for psychiatric residents in order to expose them to alternative ways of thinking based on intuitive, rather than analytical, processes. When I ran the psychiatric training program in Fresno, the faculty and I used to take the residents to Esalen for a variety of sessions in various bodywork and group therapy techniques. I felt, in particular, that there was great value in exposing them to anthropologist Gregory Bateson, who was at Esalen at the time. Although the Esalen faculty was not geared toward accommodating outside groups in this fashion, they made an exception in our case because of my connections with Michael. The fact that faculty and residents worked together as equals was good for *esprit de corps* (particularly when we all shared the nude hot tubs for which Esalen is so famous—the only problem being that my plump psychoanalyst colleague, Helen Stein, would not go in). Now that psychiatric residency has become so biological in orientation, it is difficult enough to provide adequate exposure to psychodynamic psychotherapy, let alone to experiential approaches. In addition, reimbursements to psychiatrists by insurance companies reflect their limited view of the value of psychotherapy even for psychiatric disorders, never mind its relevance to physical disease.

One individual who tried to tackle the issue of the importance of training in the psychology of the unconscious was distinguished psychoanalyst Robert Wallerstein, pioneer in research on psychotherapy and former Director of Research at the Menninger Clinic, who was Chair of the Department of Psychiatry at UCSF when I served as Vice Chair. In an effort to create autonomously functioning mental health practitioners thoroughly linked to psychoanalysis but rooted more broadly in the whole range of biological and social sciences, Bob spearheaded a Doctor of Mental Health program. The program, which fell somewhere between psychiatry and psychology, was designed to produce *partially* medically trained individuals who would serve primarily as psychotherapists but would also be able to prescribe medication. Although I was opposed to the idea, I certainly feel it preferable to the currently controversial movement to allow *completely* medically untrained psychologists to administer psychotropic drugs (as if they cannot also affect liver or kidney!). The Doctor of Mental Health program involved two years of neuroanatomy, neurophysiology, psychology, sociology, and psychopharmacology, followed by a standard, three-year psychiatric residency. The program got approval from the University of California and even produced two sets of graduates before it was killed (as a result of heavy lobbying by California's Medical and Psychiatric Associations) by state legislature disapproval of licensure for such individuals beyond the lowest level typically granted to two-year trained social workers and marriage, family, and child counselors. (Nowadays, not only psychopharmacology but also psychoneuroimmunology makes clear the value of full medical training.)

CHAPTER VI

MURDERERS I HAVE KNOWN (AND SOMETIMES LIKED)

*Of all creatures that were made, he [man] is the most
detestable . . . He is the only creature that inflicts pain for
sport, knowing it to be pain . . . Also in all the list, he is the
only creature that has a nasty mind.*

Mark Twain

My interest in criminal behavior was piqued by a variety of experiences within the criminal justice system obtained through my consulting work while I was at Stanford. (At that time Stanford did not permit its faculty to have private practices, but we were allowed to take consultation jobs one day a week.) The first of these experiences was with the California Department of Youth Authority (which, hereafter, I shall simply refer to as the "YA"), the system for handling convicted juvenile offenders. At least in those days, before becoming swamped with gang-related youths, the YA (unlike the Adult Authority, or prison system) made a genuine effort to rehabilitate many of its incarcerated young offenders. [I feel that an offender is most amenable to treatment when very young, before patterns have become ingrained, or in middle age, after antisocial behavior seems a dead end and the individual (perhaps through burnout or eventual learning by experience) begins to take personal responsibility for his behavior.]

I spent two days a month at the O.H. Close School for Boys, a new reform school for 400 delinquents in Stockton, CA, and the first of a complex of four such schools to be constructed. Being a model institution, the school was able to glean the finest staff from the entire system. The counselors took great interest in the wards, who partook of job training, education, and therapeutic programs. As one of the psychiatric consultants recruited from Stanford, I provided staff consultation, group sessions, and individual evaluation. After my colleagues and I observed that the young boys seemed to do best when identifying with an older ward who was doing well, I recommended a junior counseling program; whereby, older juveniles who were making good progress served as supervised counselors for younger wards, with whom they were carefully matched. The program was effective, and it persists to this day.

One day, an 18-year-old ward, who was serving as a junior counselor but with whom I was not well acquainted, asked me plaintively, "Doc, I've been locked up over two years this time, and I finished high school here, but I have no skills, no money, and no place to go. My father died several years ago, and my mother hasn't answered my last fourteen letters. What is going to become of me?" The boy, Jim, explained that his toughness had enabled him to survive ostracism and bullying as result of being a blue-eyed blonde in South Central Los Angeles (Watts), where he attended a 97% African-American school. I was overcome by the young man's dilemma and didn't know what to say. Serendipitously, at that time I was serving as "house shrink" to the Delta Tau Delta fraternity at Stanford. The "Delts" were a notoriously rowdy group of top athletes at the University, particularly in football. A group of Delts had once abducted a newly elected student body president at Stanford, a long-haired liberal, who later became the husband of singer, Joan Baez. (This was the '60s.) Labeled as a "hippie", he had been taken by some Delts out to the mountains behind Stanford, where they shaved his long hair and left him nude by the road. I had considered this act to be such a gross infringement of the young man's rights that I wrote an open letter to the Delts, which was published in the *Stanford Daily*. As it turned out, about half of the Delts had felt that what had happened was wrong, and the other half had felt that the "hippie radical" had gotten what he deserved. The incident and the ensuing public reaction had created such a furor within the house that the fraternity president, whom I had gotten to know the previous summer, had asked me to mediate some group meetings with members of the fraternity in an attempt to bring about reconciliation. (I had befriended the president of the Delts while vacationing with my family at Stanford Sierra Camp—a Stanford owned vacation and conference center in the Sierra Mountains. He had been the director of waterfront lakeside activities and, being water ski enthusiasts, my kids and I had become well-acquainted with him. The fall after we had met, he had been elected president of the fraternity.) The mission was successful, leading to a long-term, approximately monthly ritual, whereby I would be invited to the fraternity for dinner and a "rap" session on the topic of the day (for example, problems between the team members and the football coach).

An evening with the Delts happened to be scheduled the day after my conversation with the young man at the O.H. Close School. Breaking from tradition, I launched in with, "I don't want to hear about any of *your* problems. I'm very upset and I have a problem I want you to help me with." Telling them the story about the young man at the Youth Authority, I pressed, "An excellent junior college (Foothill) is not far from campus. I'll get him a bicycle. He can go there. You have 50 guys living in the house and plenty of extra beds, and the amount of food he eats won't even be noticed because I'm sure you throw out enough to feed one extra person." The Delts were receptive but cautious, "We certainly can't take him without meeting him." So, a defensive lineman on the Stanford football team who favored the idea, longtime buddy Jack Alustiza, was delegated to go to the reform school in Stockton to meet Jim. His report was positive, and the fraternity agreed to the experiment with the promise that I would help them deal with any problems that might arise.

A complication soon occurred. Jim was caught smoking "pot" (marijuana) and given three more months on his sentence, leading to a summer release date when the fraternity would be closed because Stanford was not in session. I arranged for a counselor to bring him to my home, where there was an unoccupied separate guest cottage. I said to my former wife (perhaps this is an example of why she is former), "If you don't want him to spend the summer with us until he can move to Stanford, you tell him because I don't have the heart to." Jim spent the summer with us, moved to Stanford, got a job as a waiter, and (after finishing junior college with excellent grades) was able, with support of the athletes, to be admitted to Stanford. I was, however, angry that there was no provision in Stanford's scholarship eligibility requirements to allow for a genuinely underprivileged student who was not of racial minority status. (Even a doctor's son had gotten a minority scholarship.) I felt it entirely unfair. Here was an impoverished Caucasian youth who had nothing. I advised Jim to use his savings, and helped him some, knowing that if he did well for one year at Stanford he would get the financial aid necessary to finish at the university (which was indeed the case). I consider Jim to be my foster son. Now fifty, he has an excellent marriage and a prospering business, based on his work as a waiter, designing and fabricating interiors for restaurants and other businesses.

In my next attempts to help such disadvantaged lads, I found that the answer was not quite so simple. I arranged for another young man from the YA, Ron, to stay at the Delts. Ron had a stormier course, but it ultimately worked out well. He is also happily married, with a child. We visit with each other whenever I am in the New England area. Ron has an identical twin brother, who has continued to be in and out of trouble his entire life. Obviously genetics isn't the whole story. A third attempt at such placement in a different fraternity was highly unsuccessful, however, in that the delinquent youth ripped off a number of the members of the fraternity. After that, I ceased my efforts to place YA kids into fraternities. Perhaps, a more formalized program with adequate supervision might have worked.

The relative success of the YA was demonstrated by research showing comparable efficacy between the programs at the O. H. Close School and the subsequently built Karl Holton School, which used different methods. O. H. Close used psychotherapeutic (individual and group counseling) approaches; Karl Holton used behavior therapy techniques (positive and negative reinforcements via merits and demerits). There turned out to be relatively little difference in recidivism between the two schools. I believe that the success of both approaches was largely attributable to the personal staff-ward *relationships*, which could not be avoided at Karl Holton as sanctions for negative behavior (that is, behavior therapy) could not be avoided at O. H. Close. Perhaps, the bottom line was that both schools were trying to help delinquent youths mature responsibly and not merely trying to punish them.

After several years with the California Youth Authority, I accepted a role as psychiatric consultant to a group home for less than two dozen delinquent teenage boys that was being set up by a Jesuit brother, who had himself come from a deprived, minority background. I relished the opportunity to work more intensively with a smaller group of delinquents. Over the considerable opposition of neighbors, a lovely home in an upper middle class section of San Jose was obtained. (The prior setting at a Jesuit monastery proved unsuitable because the rambunctious kids disturbed the tranquillity of the retreat-type setting, where semicloistered monks grew grapes and made sacramental wines.) The resistant neighbors were quickly won over by the helpful kids, who would mow their lawns and maintain their gardens (and probably helped make the neighborhood safer).

The house was staffed optimally. The counselors were generally athletes from the University of Santa Clara, who provided fine role modeling for the kids in exchange for a stipend enabling them to attend school, giving the university a better football team than usual. The home had a wonderful cook to prepare meals for the boys. There was a part-time social worker. There was I, the psychiatric consultant. The Probation Department provided one officer for the entire group of boys, all of whom had been in serious difficulty with the law and who otherwise would have gone to the YA. Fortunately, she was both competent and genuinely interested in the kids. (She and I had such a good rapport that later her son, whose private adoption I arranged, became my godson.) The chief counselor position was always filled by a caring and socially concerned male graduate student. And then there was the cleric, the full-time director who ran the place—

a remarkable and tough African-American man who went to bat for the kids, wrangling with authorities or judges as necessary. [At that time, there were very few African-American members of the Society of Jesus (Jesuits).] The boys were pretty hard core delinquents (ranging in age from 15 to 19) who did quite well, although they required a great deal of supervision. I made myself available to the staff and kids on an informal basis one entire evening a week; thus, I was not so much viewed as a therapist but as part of the "family". This system proved to work well. I could be sought out as needed, not as a "shrink". Over a period of a couple of years I witnessed some gratifying success stories—college, marriage, jobs. There were the inevitable failures as well but far fewer than expected, given my experience with the YA. The home seemed simply one of the best imaginable.

A poignant episode comes to mind. One of the older boys asked if I had some yard work that he could do to earn a bit of money. With six and a half acres, I certainly did. After my usual Friday evening dinner and rap session at the house, he rode home with me to spend the night in our guest cottage so he could work on Saturday. On the way, he begged me to stop at a bar south of Stanford in order to see his mother who was working there as a cocktail waitress. Although I was tired, I agreed. When we got to the bar, it was instantly clear that his mother was not a waitress but a hooker. She graciously introduced us to her "boyfriend", only a few years older than the kid, who was obviously her pimp. She bought me a beer and the kid a coke, chatting pleasantly before "resuming work". On Saturday, the kid did only a fraction of what I had paid him to do. As I drove him back to the house that evening, I angrily lectured him on the importance of keeping one's commitments. He began to cry, saying, "I didn't know what my mother did." (I had assumed that he had known.) I felt terrible about my own obtuseness and insensitivity. I believe that doctors should take the blame for their mistakes as well as the credit for their successes. We all make errors, hopefully not often.

One evening, the brother running the house asked me to speak individually with one of the older kids who was showing signs of significant emotional disturbance. I was shocked to find that the young man had been wrestling with the expressed emotional attachment of the director himself and corresponding sexual pressures. In worrying that this might not be an isolated case, the chief counselor and I arranged to hold a meeting of all the residents at a time when the brother would not be present (with the permission of the boy who had confided in me in the first place). The youths informed us that the director never liked to sleep alone, and so someone would sleep with him each night. Varied contact, never forceful, occurred at those times. The kids attested that they had the situation well in hand. None of them liked to do this, but since they felt to be a small price to pay for such a great living situation, they minimized their individual burden by developing a rotational duty roster. I was aghast. How could I have been so oblivious to what was going on? The many positive features of the program could not be denied. Out of respect for the brother's efforts and for him, I confronted him first. Upon hearing what I had learned, he became upset and violent. Being a physically powerful man, he threw furniture around the room, smashing a chair into many pieces against a table. He then pulled out a pistol from a drawer, pointing it at his temple. I literally got on my knees and prayed aloud for him not to take his own life—that this would be no solution to the problem. (Knowing how closely murder and suicide are linked, I was in reality scared for both of us.) He threw the gun to the floor and stormed out of the house. I learned later that he had gone to a rough, "straight" bar, where he had gotten plastered and beaten up a patron or two.

I felt that I had no choice but to report the situation to the rector of the university, a superb human being and friend, who happened to be a Ph.D. psychologist as well. He assured me that he would take care of the matter promptly and appropriately. Immediately, the director was removed from his post, and the chief counselor was made temporary director. (Not long thereafter, the brother discreetly resigned from the Jesuit order.) We soon had to face devastating news, however, that none of the other clerics at the university or in the nearby community was interested in assuming the responsibilities of a home for such difficult youngsters. (Most of the Jesuits were involved in academic or theological pursuits.) Moreover, it was the former director's motivation and energy that had been critical to the survival of the home. He had scrounged money and supplies necessary to maintain the costly operation. Within months, the home was closed, and the kids either reverted to parole on the outside, went into other group homes, or wound up back in the YA. The youngsters felt betrayed by me. I had taken their deeply valued home away from them, the best place in which they'd ever lived. They also felt that I had had no right interfering with a system which they had managed successfully on their own. They had been generally fond of the director and felt that the home was their entree to good schools, to a nice neighborhood, to security, to the comforts of a nice home, and, especially, to being cared about. As guilty as I may have felt about this at the time, I don't see how I could have turned my back on what I considered to be a completely unethical situation. What would you have done? The decision was a tough one. (These were the days before legal child abuse reporting requirements.) Amazingly, in later years, I had a friendly encounter with the former Jesuit brother. He apparently had not held against me what had transpired.

I did a short consultancy stint at a standard mental hospital in Stockton for the State Department of Mental Hygiene that ran all the public mental hospitals. It was both boring and depressing. It wasn't the patients I couldn't take; it was the staff and lack of programming. Case in point: a particularly interesting and verbal schizophrenic patient was able to explain rather eloquently his life problems and delusional ideation to me. I suggested that the ward physician, an international (new euphemism for "foreign") medical graduate with negligible psychiatric training and a relatively poor command of the English language, work with the patient individually. The physician snapped, "You academics. What use are you as consultants? Here I have 400 patients under my care, and you expect me to spend time working with a single patient?"

"Individual work with that patient may, indeed, not benefit the patient, but you owe it to your other patients to work with him for the simple reason that a patient like that can teach you a great deal about schizophrenia, about which you know virtually nothing." I certainly did not endear myself to that physician.

I promptly switched my consultancy to the more challenging Atascadero State Hospital, an institution designated for the criminally insane and mentally disordered sex offenders. The criminally insane are those too ill to stand trial (who are hospitalized until they are able to do so) and those adjudicated as legally insane. Illness criteria are highly stringent for inability to stand trial: the inability to grasp the nature of the charges or its consequences, the inability to understand the roles of the courtroom players, or the inability to participate with a lawyer in one's own defense. Although definitions of legal insanity have varied in this country, they have generally been based on the M'Naghten rule, promulgated in Great Britain over a century ago, of being able to distinguish between right and wrong and to comprehend the nature and quality of one's actions [cognitive, not volitional ("irresistible impulse") criteria].

The other 50% of the patients at this approximately 2,000-bed hospital were mentally disordered sex offenders, a very poorly defined term. This group lumped together rapists and child molesters with some nonviolent offenders, primarily exhibitionists but some voyeurs and fetishists. For example, I saw a totally harmless, severely schizophrenic young man in his 20s who had been at Atascadero nine years for having stolen a case of Coca Cola. He had been judged not guilty by reason of insanity to a misdemeanor (not felony) with a then required indeterminate sentence, not permitting release until he was "well". This young man should have been placed in an open hospital and not locked up in a maximum security hospital with murderers and rapists. Thanks in part to consultants from Stanford, the law for such offenses was subsequently changed, limiting the stay in that hospital to not longer than one could have been sentenced to jail or prison (in his case 90 days). Then there was the weird but harmless guy who did a few months of time at Atascadero after a minor traffic infraction. Being afraid of women, he had assumed the practice of being accompanied by a store mannequin, taking "her" for drives.

Sometime later, while serving on a task force of the California

Psychiatric Association, we recommended repeal of the entire mentally disordered sex offender law. Rape and child abuse are more aggressive than sexual acts and should be handled through the criminal justice system, while voyeurism, exhibitionism, and fetishism, generally can be handled as outpatient psychiatric problems. The recommendation was made with the caveat that there be special treatment programs for these people within the prison system (which was not done) and that child molesters be protected from victimization by other criminals (which was not completely done). Atascadero was a veritable gold mine of information on the criminally insane and sex offenders. Lamentably, in all its years, it had done no research on their characteristics or on the predictability of recidivism.

Prior to assuming my official consultancy at Atascadero, I had arranged through the Superintendent to get a perspective on the institution from the patients' point of view, that is, to experience criminal hospitalization first hand. (This experience was enough to cure me of the idea of a mock incarceration in prison.) I wanted to be admitted as a mentally ill patient with the story that I had threatened to kill the president (actually having hostile feelings toward him for what was happening in Vietnam). I claimed to have been working as a laboratory assistant at Stanford, figuring that the closer the story came to my actual situation, the easier it would be to pull off. My true identity would be unknown to anyone but the superintendent. He insisted, however, that I be placed among the less psychotic inmates, namely, the sex offenders. He wanted me to pose as a child molester, about which I wasn't too pleased.

I was terrified going through the usual admission procedure, being stripped down and put into a deindividualizing khaki uniform. I fantasized saying, "But I'm *really* a doctor," and getting the reply, "Sure; lots of our patients are" as a response. It reminded me of a true story about my father's former boss at Johns Hopkins, the famous American psychiatrist Adolf Meyer, whom Queen Marie of Romania had requested to meet while on a diplomatic visit in 1937. On the day of the appointment, after keeping the Queen waiting for quite some time, Meyer finally emerged. The Queen greeted him saying, "How do you do, Professor Meyer, I'm Queen Marie of Romania," to which he psychiatrically remarked, "And how long has this been going on?"

Disastrously, a shakedown yielded two sleeping pills that I had smuggled to get me through my two nights as a "patient". I was to be scheduled for disciplinary action. My pulse raced at 160 beats per minute by the time I reached the ward. The other patients clustered around me to ask what was I there for, where was I from, what did I do, how did I get caught, what was my rap, and so forth. I was stammering in the struggle to recall my prerehearsed spiel. To my amazement, one of the other patients seemed truly empathic. (A psychopath, or antisocial personality, by definition, is incapable of empathy because one cannot victimize if one can empathize.) He rebuked his peers, "Look at him; don't you see he's sweating and trembling and extremely nervous? Don't you recall how you all felt the first day you got here, how scary it was?" Next, I was briefed by the ward chief on the rules of the unit, which I was much too tense to absorb. Among those rules was never being alone in a room with one other patient. Later, the patient who had befriended me invited me for a cigarette. Being a cigar smoker, I figured I'd share a cigarette (without inhaling!) to be sociable and to express my appreciation for his thoughtfulness. He led me to his cubicle and without a moment's notice, his hand went straight to my crotch. I leapt up in terror and dashed down the hall. I was most anxious during my two nights and three days there. Unquestionably, the experience made me a more empathic consultant.

Subsequently, I went for my first consultant visit, the staff never having been informed of my experience as a "patient". I was greeted by the ward chief of a sex offender unit, a female Ph.D. psychologist clad in a khaki army blanket, out of which a hole had been cut for the neck, that draped over her dumpy figure. She inquired, "Do you want to meet the patients?" "I'd be glad to; whatever you think is best, Dr. Marigold." She proceeded to scream at the top of her lungs, "Hey you cock suckers and baby fuckers, come here and meet our new consultant!" Facetiously, I used to say that the only difference I could discern between the patients and staff of Atascadero at that time was that some of the patients got well. In that regard, it was the sickest "professional" environment I could ever have imagined with the most bizarre group of psychologists and psychiatrists I have ever encountered.

The hospital did have some redeeming qualities, however. In addition to serving sex offenders and the criminally insane, it had one ward for the most violent patients in the entire California state mental health system. This ward had double the ratio of personnel to patients than other wards (eight to 28), and the psychiatric technicians were particularly well-suited, being selected for size and gentleness. The staff would respond instantly to sudden assaults, often from brain-damaged patients, with overwhelming force applied in a humane and gentle manner.

Atascadero was very hot in the summer, and the hospital was not air conditioned. One day a 550-pound psychiatrist in his late 30s ("Dr. Humongous"), probably the most gifted and innovative of the hospital staff, collapsed at my feet, ashen and clammy, with a very rapid and thready pulse. Because of his gross obesity, I thought that he had had a myocardial infarction (heart attack). While dashing around to find a crash cart for resuscitative measures, I heard him utter, "Don't worry, I'm taking 15 grains of thyroid a day in order to reduce." (This was vastly above the allowable prescribed dosage.) For several months, this particular psychiatrist had been treating an impostor, who had successfully impersonated an Air Force colonel and a neurosurgeon. (Thankfully, he only treated back pain and other syndromes conservatively, referring elsewhere those requiring actual operative intervention.) The chronic impostor does not actually have the desire to be what he pretends to be, but gets a charge out of fooling people. Dr. Humongous devised a very clever treatment plan. The doctor himself was a rather accomplished musician, who played both drums and flugelhorn in a local jazz band. He told the patient that hospital discharge was contingent upon his becoming proficient at the drums. Given the patient's lack of intrinsic sense of rhythm, actual mastery would take time and could not be faked. Dr. Humongous also claimed that he never had to use antidepressant medication or electroconvulsive therapy with his depressed patients. Since depressed people tend to direct anger toward themselves, he would work out a routine to elicit their anger on the premise that this would relieve their depression. [Some evidence along these lines may be relevant to PNI. For example, during the Korean war, prisoners knew that when one of their compatriots gave up and crawled into a corner, he would die within a few days. Fellow prisoners would then provoke him by insulting his mother or kicking him, utilizing whatever means necessary to anger him and, thus, save his life. We had found in our Psychoimmunology Lab that mice who spontaneously develop fighting behavior have greater tumor immunity than nonfighting animals, to which they are genetically identical. My UCLA colleagues Francesco Chiappelli and Edwin Cooper showed that the *defeated* of two fighting fish develops profound immune deficiency and usually dies. (Survival of the fittest!) More recent work that I have done at UCLA with former postdoctoral fellow Volker Stefanski of the University of Bayreuth suggests that, unlike animals which fight back, those that consistently take a posture of defeat when being attacked for intruding upon a stable male-female pair show a shift in their T cell subsets and a decline in complement—a complex group of soluble blood proteins that facilitate the inflammatory immune response.] Dr. Humongous would enlist not only the staff but other patients in treating the depressed individual. His favorite method was to hand a new depressed patient a bucket of soapy water and a toothbrush, demanding that the patient scrub down the filthy walls of the ward, all the while having to endure staff and patient beratement for poor quality of work. It would take about three days for the patient to dump the bucket of soapy water on him, another staff member, or a fellow patient—at which point a marked improvement would occur.

In what proved to be my final chapter with Atascadero, I had observed one of the psychiatrists consistently demeaning and tormenting some of the patients and not ceasing despite my direct comments about his unprofessional behavior. I, therefore, reported him to the superintendent, "Dr. Mean is being abusive toward patients."

"Oh I'm fully aware of that, but he only picks on aggressive offenders. He's very nice to child molesters."

"That is irrelevant. Abuse of *any* patient is inappropriate."

"I know he has sadistic tendencies because he had a very mean father."

"Well, so did Hitler! I'm not concerned about his father, I'm concerned about the patients!"

"I know one of your concerns is that he has no criteria for the release of rapists, but I keep close track because I know when they're ready for release."

"I'd be most interested in your criteria because I find it enormously difficult to predict whether they will reoffend."

"Well, I tell by oil."

"Oil?"

"Yes. [Although this is a facsimile of the recipe, the ingredients are irrelevant.] It's two parts sesame oil, one part peanut oil, and three parts olive oil. Then the patient and I get naked, oil each other down, and we wrestle. I can tell by his response whether or not he's going to reoffend."

I reported the "oil prognosis method" to the State Department of Mental Hygiene. I got fired. The other consultants, also members of the Stanford faculty, quit. Governor Reagan then appointed a Board of Inquiry. The superintendent told them openly and sincerely about the validity of his oil method of determining the recidivistic potential of aggressive sexual offenders. Out of this inquiry came one of the most positive events of the Reagan administration in California: the firing of the *entire* psychiatric staff of Atascadero. Its very nice, sane *surgeon* was left in charge. Thus, for some time, there wasn't a single psychiatrist involved in the care of 2,000 mentally ill or disturbed patients—actually an improvement. Atascadero is *now* the best staffed mental hospital in California, with dozens of highly competent and Board certified psychiatrists, and a major source of training in forensic psychiatry for both UCSF and UCLA.

I learned the difficulty of predicting reoffense the hard way. Geoffrey was a rapist at Atascadero who had filed a *writ of habeus corpus* for his release, rendering the hospital responsible for proving why it should have to keep him. Appearing unaggressive and decent, he had been an eager participant in therapeutic activities, able to spout insights. With some reluctance to vouch for his harmlessness, I arranged for him to be transferred to the UCLA Neuropsychiatric Institute and Hospital (NPI) which, like UCSF's Langley Porter Psychiatric Institute, in those days dually functioned as a state hospital and a university teaching hospital. With state funding, these institutions could evaluate and treat particularly interesting or difficult cases from the state hospital system. A two-week evaluation at the NPI yielded the conclusion that, although they could not state so unequivocally, Geoffrey appeared to be mentally stable and probably did not represent a risk to others. He was discharged by court order.

After his release from Atascadero, Geoffrey acquired a job (with some help from me) and three girlfriends (with no help from me): an older woman, an intellectual librarian, and a sexy airline stewardess. (In my opinion, these women represented his respective desires for a mother figure, a good education, and a beautiful woman.) Nonetheless, he subsequently raped a woman whom he had just met at a bar. Following his rearrest, I interviewed all of his girlfriends, each of whom was surprised. They had all had a pleasant relationship with him with no evidence of sexual coercion or aggression. The woman Geoffrey had raped reported to me that she had refused his advances, after which he lay in wait and raped her, saying, "You don't turn me on, but your refusing me turns me on." Psychodynamically, Geoffrey was coercing affection from his withholding mother and, at the same time, paying her back for her rejection of him. I learned to be very modest in my predictions, which remain extremely difficult to make. Unfortunately, the most reliable predictor of future behavior is still past behavior.

Yet, people *do* change, and there are recovery stories. Buck (whom I had examined but never treated) was a big, burly, former football player who quite strangely got his kicks out of cross-dressing as a "bull dyke" (masculine lesbian) and picking up "femme" (feminine lesbian) partners at lesbian bars. He would then drop his jeans and say, "Surprise!" What an awful experience for his victims. Twenty years after discharge, Buck called to report how well he had been doing. Susan and I invited him over for dinner, whereupon he told us of his successful and productive career as a high level employee of a major aerospace firm—never reoffending, although never forming a lasting love relationship. Thus, recidivism is not inevitable.

After the assassinations of Martin Luther King and Bobby Kennedy, a group of senior residents and younger faculty at Stanford felt that it would be appropriate to write a textbook (*Violence and the Struggle for Existence* by Daniels, Gilula, and Ochberg). I was asked to contribute, although I felt inadequately versed on the subject except for my experiences at Atascadero. I wound up writing two chapters, "Case Studies of Violence" and "Psychodynamic Aspects of Aggression, Hostility, and Violence." (Evidently, the way to become an instant expert is to contribute to a book that is considered to be authoritative for its day. I learned more about violence *after* writing about it through being called upon as an expert witness.)

I herewith present two case studies of violence as a dramatic way of involving the reader in the complexity of medical, social, psychological, and developmental issues surrounding violent behavior: the ready availability of weapons, the nature of previolent behavior, interventions that might have averted these tragedies, and legal responsibility. The second case is most unusual in that, unknown to the defendant, the murder and immediately antecedent events were tape-recorded. The reader might at least try to understand the killers' dilemmas in an effort to discern the choice of murder as the means of resolving conflict in the face of provocation, impoverishment of coping strategies, impairment of rational thinking, and feelings of desperation and rage. In addition, these scenarios might lead to a greater understanding of the sources and perpetuation of evil.

Defendant: Rick Anderson
Male, Caucasian
28 years old, Married
Charge: First degree murder and three charges of assault with a deadly
    weapon: roving sniper, killing one woman and wounding three
    others, all strangers, during two shooting sprees three days apart.
Verdict: Not guilty of murder by reason of drug-induced insanity.
(Note: Current law would likely preclude such a verdict based on
    voluntary ingestion of those drugs.)

From the time he was 15, Rick's life could be chronicled by
antisocial behaviors, being pocked with countless arrests for a variety
of offenses, especially burglary, drunkenness, and the use and sale of
narcotics. He was a notorious "burn artist", selling bad drugs to others. The only time he had not taken drugs in 13 years was during the
first nine months of his second marriage, two years prior to the crime.
Rick ultimately reverted to ingesting 60-70 amphetamine tablets a
day because "they relieved me of feelings". In times of difficulty, Rick
would turn to his father for help, becoming enraged if help was not
forthcoming. "When I didn't get what I wanted right away, I would
get in such a rage I would vomit." Occasionally felt tender feelings
were clipped for fear of unmanliness and vulnerability; relationships
were severed as necessary to keep his feelings in check. Rick felt
isolated, even from drug users. He made his first close friendship
with a patient at a maximum security hospital for the criminally insane, who subsequently murdered a hostage in an armed escape.

Rick's father was a gambler who used gifts as a way to compensate for his chronic absence. Rick was jealous of his younger brother
and, at the age of seven, threw a ball into the street for his five-year-
old brother to chase—purposely exposing him to danger. His brother
was hit by a car, remaining unconscious for 31 days. Immediately after
the "accident", Rick went on a rampage, breaking things and tearing up
the house. He felt even more neglected by his mother after his brother

came home from the hospital. About this time, his mother started drinking and became progressively more detached from the family. When Rick was 12, he found his mother in bed with a policeman, who subsequently bribed him to remain silent. The second time that he observed his mother with this man, he told his father who seemed quite indifferent. Shortly thereafter, his mother abandoned the family.

Three years later, his mother returned. One evening, while drunk, she approached him sexually. Although there was no overt sexual contact until later occasions, he became quite disturbed at her initial attempt at seduction. "It blew my mind." Rick's first crime was committed that night. He broke into a jewelry store with a hammer and stole costume jewelry for his mother, which she accepted. From this point on, his antisocial behavior escalated, and his drug history began. Rick was horrified by but unable to free himself of his sexual desires for his mother. Often, he would encourage her into drunkenness so that sexual relations would occur.

Rick's first marriage, at age 18, was to a girl of 16. They were separated several times and finally divorced while he was in prison for burglary at age 20. He felt that his mother's meddling had ruined the marriage. While in jails and prisons, he participated in homosexual acts, causing continual inner concern about homosexuality. Approximately two years prior to his shooting spree, Rick married a woman eight years his senior. He was quite jealous of her three children by a prior marriage, finally insisting that they be sent to her former husband. The birth of their own child brought on a crisis. Rick was continually beset by murderous impulses toward the child, who was five months old at the time of the snipings.

Rick was rarely without a gun. "I've always had a thing about guns ever since my father got me a rifle when I was 13. The only time before [these shootings that] I ever shot anything alive was when I shot a rabbit, and I cried like a baby when I saw what I had done." About a year prior to the shootings, he had picked up a hitchhiker who invited him home, ostensibly to make a drug deal. They "rolled some joints" (marijuana cigarettes), drank wine mixed with gin, and "dropped a roll of bennies" (capsules of amphetamine-type drug). Rick's host showed him a .38 caliber pistol that he had stolen from a police officer, and Rick was immediately determined to own it. "I decided I was going to get it even if I had to beat him over the head." Rick offered $80 for the gun, but was turned down. The host went out for a moment. Rick took the gun and split. This highly coveted, twice stolen gun subsequently became the murder weapon.

One holiday evening after having gotten "loaded" on alcohol, barbiturates, and marijuana, Rick left his father's home and proceeded to a liquor store where he bought some gin. He went home to pick up his gun and started driving. As he drove, he shot at windows aimlessly. Later, he saw a young woman getting into her car. He shot at her, shot out a few more windows, and then went home. The morning paper reported that a woman getting into her car had been killed and that her boyfriend had been arrested for murder. Rick told his wife that he thought he had killed a woman, but she insisted that it must have been his imagination. He continued heavy amphetamine intake. Three days later, he took his gun and went driving again. "I saw two older women in a car and decided to shoot them. I thought I'd really be accomplishing something. I followed them onto the freeway. I emptied a clip into their window." He was passed by a newspaper truck, the driver of which looked at him. "I thought, 'Why is the guy looking at me?'" Rick then shot into the truck, wounding the driver. The truck followed him off the freeway; so he reloaded and emptied the gun into the truck, which drove on. Continuing to drive, Rick saw others he wanted to shoot, but there "was never an opportune moment, always another car in the way or something. It was anyone I saw, for example, a kid of 15 or 16. Then I saw this guy walking, made a U-turn and called, 'Hey!' He came up to the car and I shot him. I told him I was sorry and started crying. I went home. Throughout these shootings there was no anger; there were no feelings." When the police arrived, having traced his car, Rick denied recall of his crimes. "When it was over, I had a feeling of intense excitement, but it didn't really register that I had shot people."

When I first examined him, Rick seemed calm and composed, lacking anxiety, guilt, or any real remorse. It almost seemed as if he felt that his victims had succumbed to the normal risks of life. He appeared to be a classic psychopathic personality (sometimes called the sociopath), characterized by hedonism, impulsivity, selfishness, untruthfulness, shallowness of emotion, lack of remorse or shame, an inability to learn by experience, lack of meaningful interpersonal relationships, needs for immediate gratification, and absence of any apparent goal or life plan. During hospitalization following his trial, the drug-induced confusion, disorientation, perceptual distortions, and delusions had cleared. There was neither evidence of organic brain damage nor epilepsy; there was no evidence of schizophrenic thought disorder involving loose association of ideas, difficulty in abstract thinking, primitive logic, and idiosyncratic ideas or delusions.

In spite of his emotionless psychopathology, I intuited that Rick was somehow deeply troubled. Upon confronting him with this impression, he requested to speak with me privately. With wracking sobs and head buried in hands, he told of his incestuous relationship with his mother. "It's so horrible; it's so horrible! How can I tell you?" He had come to believe that his child was a living symbol of his incestuous relationship with his mother, since his mother and wife were confused in his mind and since he had conscious fantasies of his mother during intercourse with his wife. He had taken drugs to block these horrible images from his mind. "I just had no feelings about what I was doing."

Rick's case demonstrates how seemingly senseless attacks can at least be understood. The unstable childhood with either repeated abandonment or grossly inconsistent and impulsive behavior by both parents; strong, unacceptable, and poorly controlled sexual and aggressive impulses; and judgment-eroding addictive drugs all contributed to the killings. Rick's massive, unconscious sense of guilt over incestuous behavior may have motivated punishable behavior. The senseless shooting of strangers without any apparent emotion can be understood as a defense against and displacement of strong, murderous impulses toward the wife-mother figure and the child who represented living proof of incest. Much of Rick's behavior leading up to the shootings could be viewed as defensive, providing immediate relief of unbearable affect.

Defendant: Frank Bedsloe
Male, Caucasian
33 years old, Divorced
Charge: First degree murder: shooting to death his former wife's
husband
Verdict: Guilty of second degree murder

The case of Frank Bedsloe, a husky, intelligent, soft-spoken, 33-year-old ex-Marine sergeant, is most unusual in that the murder of his former wife's husband, Joe Levy, and the immediately antecedent events were tape-recorded. Joe, an electronics engineer, had bugged his own living room in order to obtain evidence against Frank for failure to pay child support. Due to the availability of rich autobiographical material and the tape recording of the actual murder, this case is presented in more detail.

Frank was the seventh of eight children from a poor Oklahoma family. His difficult birth was unattended (raising the question of possible brain injury). As a toddler, Frank put everything he could into his mouth, a symptom of emotional disturbance called "pica", reflecting a "starvation for love". From the age of 15 months to four years he suffered convulsions, which occurred again at the age of 10 in conjunction with a high fever and shortly after he had been hit on the head by his father. Frank was a "good child", but always felt afraid and ashamed. His history is described starkly and vividly through autobiographical notes:

"A boy should be brave. Try as I would, I could never measure up to what my parents expected. I remember feeling rejected, hurt, and confused. Most of the time I was told, 'Stop asking silly questions.' 'Go and play.' 'Don't bother me now; I'm busy.' 'Good boys don't ask questions like that.' After a while, I stopped asking questions, so the only way I could find anything out was to work it out for myself. There was no one I could turn to. I felt lost and lonely. My father worked in the oil fields and as a cotton picker and was seldom at home. My mother took in washing to help keep food on the table. Even so, I remember once I was so hungry I stole some potato peelings from a neighbor's garbage can. I felt very ashamed of it.

Some of my early memories are of my sisters beating me up. I was a weak, sickly child, small for my age until 12; so it was easy for them. They clobbered the hell out of me. Usually nobody touched one of them. I would always be the one to get the spanking. I remember a lulu of a spanking once. My sisters and I found a 50-cent piece in a mattress that was airing. We were ecstatic and went to the movies. My older brother's girlfriend claimed she had lost 50 cents, and, after furious questioning, my mother started spanking us to make us tell the truth. We were spanked with a willow switch until there were no tears left. We couldn't even speak any more; only dry sobs would come.

I certainly had a fouled-up idea of what a man should be. As a child I was taught that boys don't cry, don't show emotions, don't have feelings. What a mistaken idea! One day when I was about four, I didn't have anything to sleep in, and my mother decided I would wear one of my older sister's dresses. That was a horrifying idea. I cried and screamed and begged Mother not to make me wear the dress. I even tried to put on dirty trousers and wear them to bed. She spanked me, put the dress on me, and put me to bed. I knew I was the bad one around the house. But what had I done? What was I supposed to do? What was I supposed to be? Why was I being punished? Boys don't act like girls; boys don't wear girls' clothes. How do boys act? Are they always wrong like me?

Another important factor was my parents' inconsistencies. Many times I was told a boy acted certain ways, but when I acted that way, I was wrong. Father and Mother promised things and then went back on their word. The time my father sold my horse, after telling me he wouldn't, knocked the props from under me. My mother told me boys don't act like girls, but then she made me do girls' work. I hadn't done anything, but I was bad, bad, bad. When I tried to talk to my parents, I was shoved aside because boys aren't important. It hurt so bad to see my sisters held and loved when it wouldn't have been right to hold and love me. Oh, well, I guess boys aren't supposed to want these things. They never touched me. They used to be angry at me for getting sick. I always had the idea I was feeling bad because I was in the way. I was always afraid of new situations.

After giving much thought to the matter, I'm left with three overall impressions of my childhood: that of being always afraid and confused, that of being mostly alone with no one to talk to, that of being spanked and beaten by my sisters. I stayed pretty much to myself in school. The boys in my class didn't want to play with me because I couldn't do the same things they could. The majority of my playmates were from lower grades. One day, waiting for the bus after school, a boy a little smaller than I hunted me up and kept jumping on my back. I asked him several times to leave me alone. I couldn't get away from him. If I were sitting down or standing up, he would come behind me and jump on my back. I got him down and started choking him. Finally, two big boys pulled me off him. That scared me so much that I would go to almost any length to avoid a fight thereafter. I was afraid that I had inherited my father's temper and troublemaking nature.

I suppose I had the usual confused, mixed-up feelings as an adolescent. The only difference—that is, if it is different—was that there was nobody I could talk to or confide in. I worked most of the time and had no close school friends. The few times I tried to talk to my parents about, for instance, going to dances or dating girls, they made fun of me. (Actually, I think I denied that sort of feeling for the most part.) My sister and I would get up at four o' clock in the morning and do the chores before school. One of the milk cows was a beautiful, coal black half-Jersey, half-Brahmin. She was nervous and scared around people. When my Dad tried to milk her, she fought and refused to drop her milk. He lost his temper, started beating her with a two-by-four. She was so afraid, and all he would do was beat her.

One day we went to town to do some shopping. Daddy headed for the nearest tavern. He was really tying one on, drinking everything and anything. We were afraid to ride with him when it was time to go home, but he made us. Mother was in the car with Daddy. He hit her a couple of times on the drive. The car was weaving all over the highway. He stopped to try to buy more liquor, and, when the owner of the store refused to sell him any, he really blew his stack. He came storming out of the store, jumped into the car and almost ran head-on into a Greyhound bus and a diesel truck as we roared off on the wrong side of the highway. About a quarter of a mile farther on, he was driving much too fast to negotiate a 90-degree left-hand turn. We ran off the road into a ditch. I got a deep cut on my back. Daddy hit Mother again before he got out of the car. My glasses had been knocked off, and I couldn't see. He kept hitting Mother until he wandered off in a drunken stupor. It took three hours for the ambulance to get there. Mother was groaning in pain all the time. I wanted to help her and stop the pain, but I was helpless. I was responsible, and I couldn't do anything. It was my fault, and I couldn't do anything. Mother was mumbling and delirious. I had almost decided to try and borrow a gun and shoot Daddy so he couldn't hurt her anymore when she said, 'Frank, don't kill him.' I was surprised and thought maybe I was imagining it when she said again, 'Don't kill him.' She was groaning, mumbling, and delirious the rest of the way to the hospital.

My parents' life consisted of work and more work. I used to feel that the only reason they wanted me was that I brought home money. When I was around 14, fuzz started growing around my face. When I was standing in front of the mirror wondering if I should shave, I was trying to think of a way to ask my father if I could use his razor. Mother came in and started laughing at me and ridiculing me. God, that hurt. It seemed that I was supposed to be a man, but every time I tried to do what I thought a man was supposed to do, I was made fun of. When she told my father, he laughed too."

After high school, Frank joined the Marine Corps, where he rose to the rank of first sergeant. While stationed in Texas, Frank met Laurie. She was provocative and difficult. (During his narcoanalytic interview using the drugs sodium amobarbital and methamphetamine, a procedure to be described later, it came out that the meeting had actually taken place in a brothel, a classic "rescue" relationship.) They lived together for five months before marriage and had two daughters, plus a third by Laurie's first husband. (Frank was her fourth husband.) Two years later, Frank was sent to Korea for an 18-month period. During his absence, he had difficulty maintaining communication with Laurie and, upon his return, suspected infidelity. Laurie admitted the extent of her infidelity, involving three separate affairs. Frank assaulted his wife and then made a suicide gesture, superficially lacerating his wrists. During the separation that ensued there were continual disputes about seeing the children. On one of Frank's visits, Laurie picked up a .38 revolver:

"She pointed it at my stomach from about 10 or 12 inches away. I couldn't believe it, but her knuckles were white; the trigger was partly pulled. I saw the hammer move back a little. There was wild, cold murder in her eyes. God, that hurt! She said, 'You had better get out of here,' in a cold, feelingless voice. It would have been kinder of her to shoot. I can think of nothing that hurts as bad as seeing murder in the eyes of one you love and would die for. But there's no mistaking that look. For one who hasn't seen it, there is no way to describe it. For one who has seen it, there is no mistaking nor forgetting it. I thank God that I was so tired and so numb and my feelings were so dull that I was unaware of the full depth of the hurt."

Subsequently, Laurie married Joe Levy, a prosperous electronics engineer whose relative affluence provided well for the children. For the Levys, the continual disputes with Frank over child support payments reflected not actual need but their desire to obtain full custody of the children, although the children were fond of Frank and there had been no problems when he took the children out. Evidently, for Frank to make regular child support payments meant to accept the reality of the loss of his children and Laurie, with whom he remained obsessed. During this period of time, Frank showed some inappropriate behavior, such as appearing for a domestic military flight in full battle gear.

On the day of the murder, Frank went to pick up his daughters for an outing. As had occurred during the previous visit, Joe had planted a hidden tape recorder in his living room in order to provide court documentation of Frank's delinquency in child support. A dispute transpired among Frank, Laurie, and Joe regarding child support payments. Joe, perhaps for the benefit of the tape recorder, maintained a fairly reasonable tenor throughout most of the interaction. He hounded Frank about his commitments, however, and assailed him with the consequences of failure to maintain child support. (The tape recording had been submitted to the district attorney by Laurie in the hope that it would help put Frank in the gas chamber. The district attorney made the tape available to me under court order at the request of Frank's defense attorney.)

FRANK: If I keep making these payments, I will be in no position to help the children later. I have two choices. If I pay the—
JOE: You don't have a choice! That's an obligation. The choice is not yours. It has already been decided by the court.
FRANK: This is awfully hard for me to come up here and see someone I consider my wife.

Up to this point, Joe was setting limits on the alternatives available to Frank. Now he became very angry and screamed:

JOE: Listen, all I need is to hear about one more remark like that out of you, and I'll flatten you! Do you understand that? Laurie is not your wife, and you had better damn well understand that, Bedsloe! Now what else do you have to say, real quick?

In addition to Levy's intimidation and attack on Frank's core belief that he was still married, Laurie kept interjecting herself into the conversation in a sarcastic, provocative manner, assaulting and undermining Frank on an emotional level. She continually belittled and humiliated him:

LAURIE: Will you please be quiet! You're in my house, and I'd like to say something. You made a big point about my having spent this "lavish" amount of child support on men. The last man I went with made $1400 a month and hardly needed your piddly little bit of child support. I'm getting very weary of your coming into my house with your filthy mouth. Whenever you come up here and speak, we all get irritated and disgusted.

FRANK: You said that I saw the children in June and July. My "seeing them" consisted of seeing them twice through a screen.

LAURIE: That was your fault. You always bring along your greasy, ugly, brutish friends.

FRANK: I'll have them back before midnight Sunday.

LAURIE: I think we should have a definite time.

Further bickering regarding the children's time of return ensued. Laurie objected to each proposed arrangement:

JOE: Are you coming up to date on your payments?

FRANK: I can't until next week. The money is not in the bank.

LAURIE: I don't trust you. I never trusted you. Now you've had your little scene. You'll hear from us by Monday or Tuesday about court, definitely [to obtain custody of the children, without visitation rights].

This statement likely served to erode whatever inner controls Frank still had intact, for now he pulled out his service revolver, which he had taken from its usual place in the glove compartment of his car:

JOE: What did you pull a gun for?

CHILDREN: [Screaming] Go, go!

JOE: You pulled a gun on me here in my house? Bedsloe, don't frighten the children, for God's sake!

LAURIE: Get out of here, Frank!

The children continued pathetically screaming and pleading. Frank, usually solicitous of them, seemed oblivious to their distress and entreaties:

LAURIE: Frank, get out of here!
JOE: Laurie, take the children. For God's sake, go!
FRANK: [Calmly] Since I had to pull this, I'm afraid it's not enough this time.

Frank shot Joe four times in the chest while Laurie and the children fled from the house. It took the victim, who had fallen directly in front of the hidden microphone, about 20 minutes to die. Ghastly sounds of blood gurgling could be heard on the tape. Approximately five minutes after the shooting, Frank called the police, giving the address and saying, "I have just killed someone," in a remarkably flat and unemotional tone, as he had spoken in all his previous comments. He then waited quietly for about 10 minutes, during which time the victim was having gruesome death rattles as air was sucked through the chest wounds while he tried to breathe. The gurgles began to subside, and Frank called the police again. They arrived during his call, and Frank warned headquarters to radio the officers not to break in; nonetheless, the police forced their way into the house. Frank spoke briefly to the officers and was taken into custody, shortly after which he became mute and withdrawn, a condition clinically called catatonia.

Being unable to stand trial because of the inability to participate in his own defense (muteness), Frank was taken to Atascadero, where a three-month course of antipsychotic medication gradually transformed him into a quiet, cooperative, pleasant, and somewhat aloof patient. He had no recall of the crime or events immediately surrounding it. In what appeared to be a sincere effort to remember, he consented to a narcoanalytic interview with me, the consulting psychiatrist. In spite of the medication, Frank still had no clear recall of the actual events, indicating genuine repression. He also showed considerable evidence of bizarre thinking, reflective of psychotic thought disorder. Frank wept continuously for hours under the influence of the drugs, continually referring to how deeply he had been hurt by Laurie. He also repeatedly confused her with his mother, at times referring to the two women interchangeably. Frank assumed that because he was feeling hurt, Laurie must be feeling the same—implying their one-ness and his lack of ego boundaries. He clearly still considered Laurie his wife. He also feared for her: "Laurie gonna be hurt. Children may be, too. Laurie gonna be hurt, oh, my God! [Anxiously] That dumb girl not know what she doing. She hurt me so bad; she hurt so bad, too. Let's try to save family—children. Don't want to, must, must. Love Laurie. Oh, those dirty bastards; they don't care. He gonna shoot me." Frank also reported feeling that he was dead and that, if he had shot himself, nothing would have happened because the bullet would have gone off into space: "The papier-mâché mask above my head would have slipped back into place and covered the bullet hole."

Frank was returned to court as soon as he had recovered and stabilized enough to be able to stand trial. The court-appointed psychiatrist, Dr. Alien, diagnosed him as suffering from a psychoneurotic reaction and found him to be sane at the time of the murder; sane enough to form the specific intent to kill and to know the ramifications of the nature of his act. Nonetheless, Dr. Alien conceded that Frank's judgment was impaired by his deep reservoir of hostility toward his ex-wife, which was probably displaced upon the victim.

I testified quite differently. To me, Frank showed cognitive slippage, condensation (when one idea represents several thoughts at the same time), displacement, misidentification, lack of ego boundaries, projection (the attribution of one's own thoughts, feelings, and impulses to others), and other forms of psychotic logic. It is unlikely that these distortions were drug induced. Frank's perseveration and calm following his violent act were also evidence of psychotic dissociation of thoughts and feelings that would be uncommon to all but perhaps a hardened criminal, which Frank was not. In my opinion, Frank was legally insane at the time of the crime because his perception of the nature and quality of the act lacked contact with reality. He had felt that he and his wife were one and that they and their children were in mortal danger at the hands of the murder victim. I agreed with the court-appointed psychiatrist that Frank did have the mental capacity to form specific intent to kill; however, there was no clear evidence of conscious premeditation other than the possibility of deliberation based on a delusional interpretation of the situation. His judgment was obviously grossly impaired.

Jury trial was waived, leaving the decision to the judge. (A jury trial can be waived if both the defense and the prosecution agree that the trial will be shorter and fairer without one. About 95% of all criminal cases do not go to *any* form of trial but are either dismissed or settled by plea bargain, whereby the defendant pleads guilty to a lesser offense.) The judge found Frank Bedsloe guilty of second degree (with malice) rather than first degree (also with premeditation) murder. The tape provided rather powerful evidence that this was not a premeditated and deliberated act but, rather, one of a very disturbed man in the face of major provocation. The judge stated, "As to the defendant's insanity, unfortunately, we work within the framework of perhaps an outmoded and artificial legal structure. I do feel that the defendant at the time the incident took place—here again, I put great weight on the tape recording—was oriented to persons, places, times. I believe he knew what he was doing. I don't feel the delusion, if there was one, met the standard that I am required to apply for legal insanity under the M'Naghten rules."

Frank wrote to me from prison regarding his reactions to the trial. His letter shows the sort of repression, fragmented thought process, and bizarre ideation that he was prone to demonstrate under stress:

"I don't think anyone else but you knew I wasn't quite there parts of the time. I remember your telling the judge that I grow quieter and quieter in my circumscribed illness—as I was during most of the trial. I tried to talk to my lawyer, but I couldn't even open my mouth. I hope you know what it meant to me and means to me now to know that somebody was aware of what was happening to me. Your understanding relieved part of the helpless loneliness. I was surprised at my lack of reaction as the recording was being played. I remember nothing, didn't even recognize any of the voices. When my little girl was screaming, 'Let me go,' I got the impression that I saw an image that was threatening her and her sister with a stick or whip or something. I never heard the shots. The groans of the dying man almost tore me up. He was in such terrible pain; he hurt so badly. (And I had been told I caused it.) Poor, poor man! Poor, poor man; it didn't seem fair. Nobody ever told me you could hurt so badly after you were dead, and I had died some time before. He didn't hurt so badly as I had for so long before dying, but it was all right if I was hurt. That didn't matter; I didn't count anyway, but he hurt so much. I felt the pain with him even though I was dead, but my family is safe, family is safe. Doesn't matter I dead and still hurting; family is safe. Why hurt after dead? Go to hell, burn, is all right, can take it, family safe now, is worth pain. The pain of the dying man seemed to combine with mine, but even together the pain was much less than it had been for months, maybe years, before all this happened. Then memories of the terror, uncertainty, and pain before I died started flooding back. I felt myself slipping back into insanity. No, won't go, can't let go, too hard, too much work. Can't let go; come back, come back. Shaking, but I had made it. I hadn't gone crazy again, wonderful. As the recording went on, I remembered when the police came. I was at first glad. They were ghost police. Here, come take me away. Don't be alone when dead. Then I afraid they come to take me to burn over hot coals. Does not seem fair, but is okay. Can't last forever and ever. Family is safe, not important if I hurt, is okay. As I drifted to the door to let the police in, I floated over the body with the gun beside it. That is all I can remember of the time the recording was being played. There are no words for some of the feelings. This is as accurate as I can make it."

Frank received a short sentence and was released after about eight years of imprisonment. I received Christmas cards for a number of years, in which he told me of his new family and stable life, as a good worker, husband, and father.

The issue of insanity and legal responsibility is difficult and complex. It must be recalled that for most of his life Frank Bedsloe was a hard-working, productive citizen. He was devoted to his family and had not been violent, antisocial, or overtly psychotic. One sees a man who in childhood was deprived of affection, shamed for being a male, and repeatedly the victim and witness of violence. In all these circumstances, one can sense the great pain of Frank's helplessness in doing anything about his plight. He could not help his mother after the accident; he could not prevent being forced to wear a dress; he could not stop his sisters' violent treatment of him. He expressed this great emotional pain in his letter: "The pain of the dying man seemed to combine with mine, but even together the pain was much less than it had been for months, maybe years, before all this happened." Given all this, it is not difficult to imagine how the divorce from his wife became an intolerable burden for Frank to bear or how murder could be seen as a desperate solution to an unbearable conflict.

Violence, like physical illness, has multifaceted origins: genetics, previous life experiences, current pathogenic influences, and resistance or "immunity" to such influences. What particular forces congeal to allow hostile feelings to be actively taken out on others? As I explained before, children whose aggression is *either* overcontrolled *or* overindulged cannot develop a tolerance for frustration, and they may be predisposed to later explosive breakthroughs. Cultural and social factors can encourage aggression. (In war, "rational" and impersonal killing occurs to resolve *social* rather than personal conflict.) Sometimes the victim is a scapegoat, a substitute for the person who engendered the hostility. Even among lower animals, displacement of aggression is seen. A dominant male monkey teased by a human may attack subordinate members of his group. In comparative biology, instinctual aggression promotes survival of the fittest with consequent genetic benefits. Although animals tend to attack when frustrated or frightened, their aggressive behavior alters with changes in order of dominance. Even innate animal behavior is modifiable. A wild horse can be broken to the saddle. Rats need to have had the experience of being mothered to be able to nurse their young. A female infant monkey deprived of a mother will become a hostile and abusive parent. Mice reared in a barren environment are timid about exploring new environments; whereas, those repeatedly exposed to new objects are bold and adventuresome later in life. Likewise, the control of anger in humans must be learned during development, largely through parental example. To children, actions speak louder than words. This split in ideation and behavior is illustrated by a thug who reported to me a "great admiration" for Albert Schweitzer. The psychopath is acutely sensitive to hypocrisy. He believes actions, not words. So often has he seen persons significant to him say one thing and do another that he comes to believe only what he sees, not what he hears. Insecurity stemming from inconsistent parental behavior (for example, "Do as I say, not as I do"), early deprivation of significant loved ones, parental discord, and frequent changes of residence in childhood are common backgrounds of violent persons. In particular, there is documentation of absence, death, brutality, or passive uninvolvement of the father in the past histories of male criminals and psychopaths. In my own studies of murderers, particularly mass murderers, parental brutality or sadism (not necessarily physical) were the two consistent historical features.

Both novelty and familiarity are sought by higher organisms; the balance between the two is related to prior experience and, possibly, to genetics as well. Past or current uncertainty may enhance seeking the familiar. The familiar that is sought by humans may be tumultuous and violent if one's earlier experience has been chaotic or abusive. Even in the primate world, the frightened infant monkey relentlessly seeks out and clings to a hostile, abusive mother. Thus, seemingly irrational and unrewarding behavior is a mechanism to provide certainty and security, ingredients essential to existence. It is well-known that criminals tend to stick to the same sorts of crimes. Forgers remain forgers; second-story men remain second-story men. Child psychologists have noted that children find comfort and a sense of active control through repetitive play patterns, which serve to reduce anxiety.

A hostile, punitive, and constantly critical parent who provides no praise may promote aggressive behavior by instilling in the child the belief that, "I guess I don't think *anything* I do is wrong because I really think *everything* I do is wrong." (Genuine acceptance of this belief may lead to self-loathing, depression, and suicide.) Furthermore, a parent may ignore a child except when he or she is being "bad", attention being an extremely important motivation for behavior. Once labeled "bad", a rejected child may be invested in continuing to behave destructively lest the reality of his parent's absolute uninterest be confirmed, a fact that would be too painful to face. At least, he can retain hope of being loved were he only good. Self-image may also provide a link between organic and psychological factors in the causation of antisocial behavior. The child who is impulsive, hyperactive, or destructive as the result of brain damage or dysfunction is often labeled as "bad". Although the original behavior was largely involuntary, perpetuation can result from the individual's perception of himself as evil. Freud pointed out that some people do not feel guilty because they are criminals but are criminals because they feel guilty.

Punishment-seeking behavior may serve to assuage feelings of guilt. The criminal tends to leave clues, to confess, to seek punishment. Since the unconscious operates on the principle of "an eye for an eye and a tooth for a tooth", violence may be a means to provoke punishment. The person who seeks punishment by society may be symbolically seeking the parent who spanked him. Some may murder to invoke capital punishment—a powerful argument that I have made against the death penalty.

Behavior that seems defiant (even in the eyes of the perpetrator) may actually be compliant with a parent's unconscious wishes, which are received by the child as subtle commands. For vicarious gratification, the parent gets the child to do what he or she would have liked to have done. The father of an eight-year-old arsonist, one of the youngest children ever committed to the California Youth Authority, broke into a smile and chuckled with delight as he told me of an earlier incident in which the boy had attempted to assault his younger brother with a meat cleaver, implying "That's my boy!" Unconsciously, a mother can encourage aggression in her son in an effort to bring out traits corresponding to her ideal of the masculine image or encourage promiscuity in her daughter to deal with her own sexual frustrations.

Helplessness in getting basic needs met seems to be at the core of paranoia (excessive or irrational suspiciousness of others), which often underlies individual and mass aggression. Violent coercion is a decisive way to have impact upon a world perceived as unresponsive and oppressive. The doer feels master of his own fate. The tape-recorded murder was a classic case of paranoid entrapment in which Frank Bedsloe felt that he had been reduced to one option. Both the ghetto dweller, who feels impotent in effecting social change, and the student, who has no voice in a huge bureaucratic university, may riot in frustrated, angry response to a sense of futility and powerlessness. Helplessness is sometimes manifested in grandiosity and power seeking, that is characteristic of individuals like Adolf Hitler or the schizophrenic who takes on the persona of Jesus Christ.

An evermore prevalent cause of crime is narcotic addiction, that occurs in individuals who are battling anxiety, depression, low self-esteem, and high dependency needs. Addictive drugs such as alcohol, amphetamines, and barbiturates tend to erode inner controls, judgment, and contact with reality. Since drugs can virtually dissolve conscience, they become a means to remove guilt, avoid conflict, suppress undesirable thoughts and impulses, and provide forbidden satisfactions. In reality, however, they create new problems. Stimulant drugs such as amphetamines and cocaine can actually produce paranoia of varying duration. Sedative drugs can disinhibit otherwise controlled aggressive or sexual impulses.

Different kinds of violent behavior indicate different emotional needs in the perpetrator. In sadism, pleasurable or sensuous perceptions are merged with the act of inflicting harm on another, which disguises the motivating anger or rage. This disguise prevents guilt or fear of retaliation. Masochism has been termed "the act of loving a sadist". Masochists endure abuse, injustice, and suffering not only for atonement but also as a way to bribe love or gain pity as a substitute. This suffering helps to reduce guilt and the desire for parental love. Since sadism and masochism have similar roots, they are frequently interchangeable; the tormented easily becomes the tormentor. Rape combines aggressive and sexual drives, which ethologists have noted are only precariously separated in the animal kingdom (fighting and mating). A submissive sexual posture may abort attack in animals. Since slang and folk expressions provide clues to unconscious associations, it is noteworthy that the terms "screw" and "fuck" are used interchangeably to describe sexual intercourse and interpersonal hostility. A child observing parental sexual relations often interprets intercourse as assault, a possible common basis for later sexual inhibitions. Motives of power, control, and even destruction can meld with sexual wants.

Accordingly, an act of rape may represent unconscious retaliation against parental rejection or hostility, and simultaneous gratification of needs not met. Using force can also be a means to extract love that is perceived as unlikely to be freely given, that is, "I'll never get what I want unless I take it". Murder, which sometimes accompanies rape, may signify "I punish to avoid being punished".

First-degree murder, as defined by most states, is murder that is premeditated (even by only a few moments), or deliberated upon in advance. Second-degree murder involves willful killing with malice aforethought. Legally, malice has been poorly defined. Not long ago, it was defined as "killing with an abandoned and malignant heart". (I used to like to ask attorneys to explain what that meant.) Malice is now defined as existing when killing results from an intentional act, the natural consequences of which are dangerous to human life and known by the killer, as in the case of Frank Bledsoe. Voluntary manslaughter, entails unlawful killing without malice, as in drunk driving. Involuntary manslaughter is essentially the result of an accident due to one's own negligence, such as leaving a loaded handgun in a place accessible to a small child. Homicide in self-defense is not considered a crime at all. In order to prove murder in the first or second degrees, one has to know what the mental condition of the person was at the time. The mental inability to premeditate, deliberate, or harbor malice is referred to as "diminished capacity". Many attempts to claim diminished capacity have been based upon intoxication. Since many crimes are perpetrated under the influence of alcohol that provides false courage (disinhibition), such a defense may be inappropriate. On the other hand, some intoxications [such as with phencyclidine (PCP) or LSD] can produce a psychosis or delusion and impair contact with reality. Only about one percent of homicide defendants nationwide are found "not guilty by reason of insanity". After the Dan White case (to be described), the California Legislature forbade psychiatrists to *conclude* whether "diminished capacity" existed. Nevertheless, in "specific intent" crimes, when a person's mental intent is built into the legal definition of the crime, psychiatric opinion about such states cannot really be excluded.

In California (laws in other states vary), capital punishment for first degree murder is only permissible under "special circumstances" such as those in which murder involves multiple victims, torture, killing for hire, kidnap, or rape. (Federal capital offenses include other violations such as treason.) I have argued that the *seeking* of capital punishment by a murderer is a potent argument against the death penalty. To illustrate, I testified at the murder trial of a live-in babysitter who suffocated and cut up her two young charges, of whom she said she was fond, in a conscious attempt to invoke the death penalty. She had failed several attempts at suicide and believed that her death could only be accomplished by receiving capital punishment. The death penalty is justified primarily on the basis of its alleged effectiveness as a *deterrent* to murder. The deterrence argument, however, is based on the premise of a "reasonable man". The vast majority of killings are "crimes of passion", rooted in psychopathology and not subject to rational thinking. There are no data showing that capital punishment serves as a deterrent. The elimination of capital punishment in individual states has neither increased murder rates nor has the reinstatement of the death penalty decreased them. The legitimizing of capital punishment symbolically renders society a brutal parent who uses violence as a means of coping. Since violence begets violence, we should expect, therefore, that those who live in a society that inflicts the death penalty would be more likely to choose murder as a means of problem solving.

Although I am pro-choice concerning abortion, I don't believe that any human being has the right to choose whether another person lives or dies. Actually, I cannot understand the inconsistency of so many who are both "pro-life" (antiabortion) while strongly "anticrime" (in favor of long prison sentences and capital punishment), since if any one factor relates to subsequent criminal behavior, it is being *unwanted* (not the same as being unplanned). I believe that, after having a year to think about it, a murderer could perhaps be given the option to *choose* the death penalty as an alternative to life without possibility of parole. There is, however, one condition under which I believe that capital punishment, or any killing for that matter, can be justified: self-defense. (By this standard, World War II was justified;

Vietnam was not.) Two possible "legitimate" capital punishment candidates come to mind: a person already imprisoned for life without possibility of parole who kills a guard or fellow inmate, and a terrorist, whose compatriots threaten to take hostages or kill others unless he is released. If the death penalty must exist, it should be promptly administered, and appeals should be limited. Both the costs and inhumanity of keeping people on death row in a continual state of uncertainty would then be minimized. Capital punishment cases are so costly (with unlimited fees for attorneys and experts, at least in California), even for the initial trial let alone the appeals, that it is cheaper to keep murderers in prison than to kill them.

The following case is intended to illustrate further the problems inherent in the death penalty. I testified at the trial of Chester Caldwell, a 25-year-old Vietnam veteran, who killed a drug dealer of another city for a nominal cash payment on contract. Chester had been both numbed and traumatized by the authorized killing of people in Vietnam. He felt that his offenses against society warranted his death *at the hands of society.*

Defendant: Chester Caldwell
Male, Caucasian
25 years old, Separated
Charge: First degree murder with special circumstances: killing for hire
Verdict: Voluntary manslaughter.
(Note: One law textbook subsequently referred to this unusual case as the "Manslaughter-for-Hire Case".)

Chester Caldwell, a 25-year-old, separated white man, executed a contract to kill a drug dealer of another city for a payment of $120, with $30 payable upon "delivery". The individual who had put out the contract had allegedly been ripped off by the victim who had also killed a friend of his. Chester was selected for the job because, according to the "contractor", "I know violence doesn't mean much to you." The man who had arranged their meeting was subsequently caught and turned state's evidence (agreeing to testify against his codefendants for a lesser sentence), leading to their arrest. My informants were Chester and his intelligent, perceptive, well-adjusted, married sister, Mary.

Chester's mother was a rather lenient, ineffectual, and probably masochistic woman, as evidenced by two marriages to sadistic men. His father was extremely controlling, rejecting, erratic, and cruel. Chester was a somewhat withdrawn child who tended to live in fantasy; for example, acting out the role of being a protective big brother but showing no special interest when his sister was actually sick. The father, an ex-Marine, only showed pride in Chester over two accomplishments: his being in Little League baseball, which was disrupted by an injury resulting from sticking a key in a light socket, and his joining the Marines. The achievement of long-sought-after approval and reconciliation with his father as a result of joining the Marines was aborted, however, by his father's sudden death from a heart attack while Chester was in basic training.

Prior to entering the service, in spite of difficulties with his father, Mary describes Chester as having been patriotic, generous, well-liked, and particularly helpful to others, although having a tendency toward rages. Chester joined the Marines at age 17, getting into a number of scrapes and then going AWOL because of being homesick for his girlfriend. Upon returning, at age 18, Chester was sent to Vietnam as an alternative to the brig. There he learned to kill. "The only thing is to keep yourself alive. Fuck everybody else." He served in the infantry in the most difficult combat situations, the sort of action seen by fewer than 10 percent of those who served in Vietnam.

Chester extended his enlistment for six months in order to get an early discharge with the promise of having a different military occupational specialty. The agreement was reneged upon, however, and he was kept in a line company. During the great North Vietnamese Tet Offensive that marked the turning point of the Vietnam War, his outfit replaced one that had been wiped out. "They just kept sending in guys to be killed." During the first four days of combat at Hue, the unit was restricted to the use of small rockets in an effort to preserve the ancient city. After two weeks of combat, his company had been reduced from 180 men to 40 men. While in Vietnam, Chester began to use drugs, progressing from marijuana to heroin, although he never established a physical addiction.

Chester changed after the action at Hue. He shot a Vietnamese person running out of a doorway without bothering to determine if it was a man or a woman. "It was just too much of a hassle." He had killed a pregnant girl of about 18. "I just knocked her down because she was there. I didn't care anymore. My attitude toward violence had changed; doing violence was the easiest way out of a problem. Just shoot them." When the girl's mother came out of the house screaming, she, too, was "greased". From then on, Chester wanted "to just fix it so they leave you alone—no arguing." It "became easier all the way around" just to kill. "I didn't even feel bad about it at the time. I just pushed her to the side and shoved her mother into the doorway." On another occasion, he shot an old man in the feet. After losing so many friends in combat, Chester decided that he would not make any more friends. He was tired of hearing his friends screaming in pain when wounded and his own being unable to help them without endangering himself. "I got to where I wouldn't make friends because it might involve risking my ass. On top of everything else, who needs a guilty conscience?"

Chester seemed peculiar when he returned from Vietnam. His sister felt that he was trying to act the head of the household. He would bring rowdy friends home, behaving like the "cock of the roost". Chester was very concerned with issues of power and control, getting upset, for example, when he found that his sister was driving his late father's sports car. He could not reestablish a relationship with his mother, who had remarried a dominating and jealous man. He was also unsuccessful in terrorizing his sister, who was protected by her six-foot two-inch boyfriend, whom she eventually married.

For a while, Chester hung around the house, not doing anything but drinking more and more heavily. His longtime girlfriend, now wife, Pam, was extremely compliant and probably masochistic (like his mother). Whatever he did would be all right. He treated her badly. He squandered money and alienated all of his friends. Chester had married Pam, against the objections of her parents, after she became pregnant. During the delivery of their child, he reported no feeling for her pain. He took no responsibility for the baby whatsoever. Pam went to work after the baby was born. She would get up at 5 AM, clean the house, drop the baby off at a sitter's, and go to work. They lived in poverty. Chester continued to have fantasies of violence. "When a person is dead the problem is over." Because of his in-laws' increasing objections to their daughter's unsatisfactory marriage, he engaged in continual fantasies of killing them, even though he realized intellectually that their concerns had legitimacy.

Chester reported an incident in which he and Pam had come across a freeway accident in which some children had been trapped in a burning car. Pam had become extremely upset at the grisly sight while Chester reported, "it didn't bother me a bit." He sensed that he had lost his ability to have emotions. At times, he had flashbacks in which he became frightened and required Pam to lie still on the floor with him as if they were under fire. At the time of the birth of their second child, whom Pam had wanted in order to strengthen the marriage, Chester did not even accompany her to the county hospital. She finally left him after he lost control and struck her in the face. She had become quite frightened of him. His sister, to whom he continually returned in a dependent and ambivalent way, had also become frightened of him and would have nightmares of his killing her. Mary went into psychotherapy, giving her a better understanding of her family and what had happened to Chester.

Chester recalled having been a sentimental individual prior to going to Vietnam. Since then, he no longer had the capacity to cry or to feel tenderness, except for some sense of attachment to his wife. His sister believed that he routinely went out of his way to provoke rejection. Chester was obsessed with feelings of guilt. "My country and I fucked over those people. Imagine foreign people coming and dragging you out of your own house, burning it down, and destroying everything you had in the world! I learned that if people are annoying you, you just pull the trigger Calley is no freak; that happened every day." (Chester was referring to a highly publicized case in which an officer had commanded his troops to massacre hundreds of civilians, an instrumental factor in the shifting of the American attitude against the war.) Chester was beset by continual memories of old Vietnamese ladies being tortured, picking up dead bodies, a companion who performed cunnilingus on a three-day-old legless corpse after shaking off the maggots. He had fantasies of returning to Vietnam with $1,000,000 and giving it to the people to apologize. "The United States should be on its knees trying to make up to those people."

During the year and a half after separation from his wife, Chester remained drunk all the time. He told his sister, "I'm too much of a coward to commit suicide. I'm going to do it the hard way." He was angry with his family for continuing to see his ex-wife and children. He was afraid of remarrying. "I was scared I would start blowing people away." On the other hand, "I kept hoping a situation would arise so I could take out my frustrations. A walking time bomb would have been an apt description of me." Chester was grateful when the opportunity to take a contract arose. Not only would it relieve his frustration to kill someone, but the money might enable him to get out of the city, move away from people, go to the country. Chester felt no guilt about the murder. "He was lucky; I could have made it rough for him like I was asked to." Chester had been unable to smash in the head of the dead body as requested because it reminded him of the "spookiness of the bodies in Vietnam".

Chester responded to his arrest with great indifference, "I don't care what happens, life for me is like a jail anyway." He refused to obtain or talk to an attorney, *requesting* the death penalty after a plea of guilty to first-degree murder under special circumstances (killing for hire). Finally, he accepted counsel on the insistence of his family. Chester reflected, "I don't know if I would be of any use to society as a functional human being. I don't think I could ever get over my indifference to violence. Something might come up and I would be off. I have been punishing myself since I have been back from Vietnam. Maybe it is better to go through anguish than to get disattached."

Chester Caldwell was convicted of *voluntary manslaughter* (unlawful killing, no malice). To my knowledge, after considerable inquiry, this is the first time in American jurisprudence that such a verdict was obtained in a case of killing for hire. (One juror was a Vietnam veteran and another was a psychology student.) The prosecution had confidently expected a first-degree verdict, which likely would have led to the death penalty. A lawyer facetiously referred to it as "the manslaughter for-hirecase."

CHAPTER VII

THE PRACTICE AND MALPRACTICE OF CRIMINAL JUSTICE

What win I if I gain the thing I seek?
A dream, a breath, a froth of fleeting joy.
Who buys a minute's mirth to wail a week?
Or sells eternity to get a toy?
For one sweet grape who will the vine destroy?

William Shakespeare

Just on the heels of my decision to leave Stanford in the hope of being able to start my own program, a job offer came from a most unlikely place: the County Mental Health Department in Fresno, a provincial city in the heart of California's agricultural Central Valley. In the wake of deinstitutionalization, under the leadership of Trevor Glenn, M.D., Fresno had developed the best community mental health system in the state. It offered a broad range of services—halfway houses, day care, an acute inpatient unit, outpatient services, crisis intervention, a residential living facility (a converted old motel with a resident social worker for people making the transition from institution to community), and rural outreach programs (recreational vehicles fixed up as office suites that traveled to tiny communities in the county). Fresno offered me an impressively well-funded opportunity to develop not only a residency training program but also a model treatment program for criminal offenders, under the joint auspices of the Health, Probation, and Sheriff's Departments. (At that time, the State of California had an excellent policy whereby any county that referred fewer people into the state prison system than would be expected, given its prior record of felony convictions, would receive half of the money that would otherwise have been spent on incarceration for the development of innovative prevention programs.) Moreover, I found out that the University of California, San Francisco, where I had done my psychiatric training and still had some positive connections, was going to open a branch medical school in Fresno, largely for primary care training. It was intended as a possible forerunner for a full university campus in Fresno, now actually under development in nearby Merced.

It was an offer I could not refuse. If I couldn't change the nature of medical care based on the understanding of intrinsic links between biology and psychology, I could perhaps fundamentally change criminology. (This rather grandiose goal turned out to be quite unrealistic but one which at least netted some positive outcomes. Jolly West helped me out by giving me an interim academic appointment at UCLA until UCSF officially began its Fresno-Central San Joaquin Valley Medical Education Program, which thrives to this day. It wasn't long after I began the Fresno program that I became Vice Chairman of the Department of Psychiatry at UCSF. I also served as Chief of Psychiatry at Valley Medical Center of Fresno, the county hospital.

I began by recruiting additional faculty members: among them, psychoanalyst Helen Stein of Columbia University, the best teacher of psychodynamics and psychotherapy that I have ever met. Helen was a devout Freudian, who would become incensed at any attempt to limit the relevance of psychoanalysis by placing it in the context of turn-of-the-century Viennese Jewish culture, arguing vociferously, for example, that the Oedipus complex (in which the child is intrinsically attracted to the parent of the opposite sex and feels rivalry with the parent of the same sex) is biologically determined and has nothing to do with culture. She was also a rabid atheist, in spite of (or perhaps because of) the fact that her father was an Orthodox Jewish rabbi. Psychoanalysis was Helen's religion as well as profession. (Much to her chagrin, her own children ritualistically followed the religious tradition of her father—possibly rebelling against the rebel) Helen had begun her career as a general practitioner and was able to combine biologic and psychodynamic approaches to psychiatry. The short, plump psychoanalyst with the New York accent responded characteristically to my invitation to join the faculty and participate in research on the treatment of criminals, "What do I know about psychopathy? All I know about is middle class, Eastern, intellectual neurotics." (She really knew lots more.)

Another unusual faculty member that I recruited was Danish psychologist-psychoanalyst, Claus Bahne Bahnson. Claus had done some fascinating, albeit controversial, research on the psychological characteristics predisposing individuals to the development of cancer, that later stimulated my thinking on the topic and led to his inclusion on the PNI Task Force at UCLA. Claus did a superb job in setting up training, particularly in family dynamics, for family practice residents. Appropriately, Claus later attempted to integrate psychodynamic theory into psychoneuroimmunology; however, he had difficulty relating to the more biologically-oriented individuals in the field. I agreed with his fondness for "projective" psychological testing (for example, the Rorschach "ink blot" and Thematic Apperception Tests) that reveal more of unconscious processes but which are now so rarely used in psychobiological research. Claus currently practices and heads the Psychoanalytic Institute in Kiel, Germany.

Before instituting the Model Treatment Program for Criminal Offenders, I felt it appropriate and potentially helpful to visit two of the very few purportedly successful treatment programs for criminals. One was in the Netherlands, the other in Denmark. Both were impressive, elaborate, intensive, and long programs, particularly the one at Herstednester, Denmark, run by psychiatrist Georg Stürup since the 1940s. Dr. Stürup's optimism had an important influence on me. In his book *Treating the "Untreatable"* (1968, he wrote, "Despite the inmate's own and other people's expressed opinions to the contrary, we have shown that about 90 percent of our supposedly hopeless people are capable of giving up a life of crime."

I also visited a highly controversial American attempt at rehabilitative treatment, the Patuxent Institution in Maryland. Criminals could be committed there on indefinite sentences, release being dependent upon behavioral criteria for rehabilitation. In order to be discharged, an inmate had to progress from an extremely restrictive, privilege-lacking first level to a virtually unrestricted seventh level through demonstrating ever-more-socialized behaviors. If one did not change, one could remain at restrictive levels "forever". Actual therapeutic programming was unimpressive, but one had to "shape up" in order to "ship out". Ultimately, the program was found to be unconstitutional, since the punishment fit the criminal, not the crime. Long incarceration for relatively minor offenses was found to violate the Constitution's prohibition of "cruel and unusual punishment". In reality, however, Patuxent had lower recidivism than standard prisons.

Simultaneous with the development of the Model Treatment Program, we established a good training program for psychiatric residents and a psychiatric clerkship for UCSF medical students as well. (The reputation of the clerkship was such that at one point almost half the junior class of UCSF requested to come to Fresno—a location nearly 200 miles away.) The Model Treatment Program was housed in a maximum security area of the Fresno County Jail. Twenty to 30 male inmates were involved in the residential program at any one time.

These inmates stayed in a dormitory-style setting with a comfortable dayroom area. Each had a small area of personal turf which he could decorate as he pleased; educational materials and recreational equipment were available. Program participants were either repeat offenders permitted by the judge to have a go at treatment in lieu of reincarceration in prison for offenses of moderate severity, or for those who had been given full year jail sentences. (Candidates were referred by the court for consideration and not sentenced to the program.) Recidivists and older prisoners were especially included on the premise that those beginning to realize the natural history of a criminal lifestyle would be more likely to be ready to abandon it. Naively, at the outset, I had wanted to exclude the mentally ill and drug abusers because this was not a psychiatric or substance abuse rehabilitation program: it was an attempt to deal with antisocial criminal behavior. Although we were able to eliminate at least the grossly mentally ill, it turned out that 80% of the prisoners had problems with drugs.

We used a modified version of a therapeutic community model developed in the 1950s by psychiatrist Maxwell Jones of Great Britain, which had been shown to be relatively effective for psychiatric problems manifested primarily through acting out (not for schizophrenia, as it was often mistakenly assumed). His model utilized joint committees of staff and participants for decision-making by consensus; ours made decisions by majority vote. In light of the fact that the professional staff bore the ultimate responsibility for carrying out group decisions, we also gave our staff veto power over community decisions (although rarely was this necessary). Acceptance to the unit, disciplinary action, ejection from the unit, and promotion to greater levels of responsibility were all determined by staff and clients together. (We did not refer to the inmates as patients because they were not mentally ill.) Progressive levels of responsibility included: supervised offsite athletic and recreational activities, trusteeship (an unpaid junior staff position in the prison with special privileges), home visits, and work furlough.

Ultimately, the staff grew to include part-time psychiatrists, a psychiatric resident, probation officers, sheriff's deputies, a social worker, and an ex-convict worker, all selected for humaneness. Emotional maturity, some college education, psychological-mindedness, warmth, and likeability were strong prerequisites for correctional personnel. We were fortunate to have, as head of correctional personnel, a dedicated and well-educated sheriff's sergeant with an outstanding record in civil rights, who was respected by both the inmate population and his superiors. The team's most valuable player, however, turned out to be the explicitly sought ex-convict. Thirty-six-year-old Doug had served 10 years in prison and had been crime-free and productive for over eight years. Doug had had experience with Synanon (a self-sustaining community designed for rehabilitation of convicts and drug addicts that eventually became involved in criminal activities, led by the charismatic Charles "Chuck" Dietrich). Just as recovered alcoholics are indispensable to alcohol treatment programs, the ex-con provided a more realistic, unthreatening role model, and his knowledge of the prison subculture made him difficult to con. Rehabilitated former convicts with appropriate training can be effective staff members, but only one or two should be on the staff of any unit. Excons, on the one hand, tend to overidentify with the prisoners and, on the other, can be more punitive than other members of the staff.

An essential part of the program was small group therapy, co-led by correctional officers and mental health professionals. These sessions, along with community meetings, aided conflict resolution and group cohesion. In the small group setting, evasions were quickly spotted by participants, and socialization pressures were intense enough to foster relatedness and, thus, acceptance, trust, and sometimes affection. Each prisoner was assigned a psychiatrically supervised counselor to serve as advocate, therapist, role model, and confidante. Insight-oriented, traditional psychotherapy was offered individually to the few who seemed to have amenable psychopathology and motivation. Conjoint interviews with family members were held whenever possible. Unfortunately, most did not have intact or cooperative families.

I resisted using confrontation techniques that had been applied rather successfully in the original Synanon residential treatment program and, later, in the far better Delancey Street program. This technique is a sledgehammer approach to breaking down psychological defenses. (Any willingness on my part to consider using these techniques was predisposed from my medical school days, when I witnessed my gentle and kind father, in consulting for the Air Force, call an airman a "chicken shit wimp" for not having the strength to face the fact that behind his tough bravado he was actually a scared kid. The airman actually sobbed. Although at the time I had thought that Dad was being mean, later I saw how necessary it was for the airman to come to grips with his pattern of acting out conflicts and blaming others.) My real problem with confrontation techniques, however, was that breaking through defenses to access deep-seated insecurities and feelings, such as abandonment, hurt, and worthlessness, seemed hardly adequate in and of itself. Therefore, ours was a double whammy method. We used the sledgehammer of confrontation to uncover conflicts, fears, and vulnerabilities and used traditional, largely group, therapeutic methods *to work on them.*

I recall the first time that Helen Stein ever made a confrontation at one of our community meetings. Each time she tried to say anything, she was shouted down by a very aggressive, six-foot six-inch, muscular African-American man. Finally, the five-foot three-inch Helen rose to her full height and screamed in her New York accent, "Pawul, Pawul (Paul)! Goddammit! Stop trying to shove your cock down my throat!" That stopped Paul, and Helen was listened to thereafter. One of my favorite psychiatric residents of all time was a lovely, dignified, and reserved woman of German origin by the name of Rosemary, who also had problems similar to Helen's in the confrontation group. (Rosemary was somewhat older than the average resident because she had decided to become a psychiatrist after having practiced internal medicine and raised a family for a number of years.) When first assigned to this unit, she was continually reduced to tears by these aggressive men. I finally suggested to Rosemary that, in light of the facts that most residents do not train in settings like this and that she planned to go into private practice, I thought it would be best to place her in another rotation at no penalty to her training status whatsoever. She responded thoughtfully, "You're probably right, but I hate to admit defeat, so let me try it here for another couple of weeks." Shortly before her two weeks were up, as she was being attacked once again, she gave her attacker the finger, shouting, "Up yours, you motherfucking, cocksucking punk!" He shut up and Rosemary, too, was thereafter accepted by the community. After the meeting, the devoutly Catholic Rosemary said, "I never believed I could ever say such words in my life." Her psychiatrist husband subsequently called me, inquiring, "What are you doing to Rosemary? She's getting so assertive at home!" Rosemary wound up doing a wonderful job and learning a great deal from the Model Treatment Program.

I made errors myself in learning to deal with criminal psychopaths, one of my most painful lessons occurring during a weekend marathon confrontation group. Feeling tremendous pressure and not wanting to chicken out, I allowed myself to be in the "hot seat". After being badgered relentlessly by the group for hours, I finally opened up somewhat personally. The immediate effects seemed good, and I felt more warmly and humanly accepted, but what I had revealed was later used against me. Helen had advised nonparticipation to maintain more therapeutic distance. She was right.

I literally nearly gave my life for the Model Treatment Program and inadvertently made a significant discovery about psychophysiology, the ability of the mind to exert control over bodily functions. A hit man was sent to kill me by a former client of the program, a Mexican-American named Luis, who had been voted out of the unit for nonparticipation. After being voted out, Luis spoke to me privately and disclosed that he had a problem with impotence. I explained to him that, had he still been a member of the community and not been awaiting transfer to prison, we should have at least made an attempt to help him with that problem, although I was not sure if we could be of any help. He then told me that when he was "fucking a guy", he would fantasize "being fucked".

"Well, perhaps that has something to do with your problem of impotence."

"Don't you think I don't know that? I'm not stupid!" (In prison culture, one is not considered homosexual as long as one is the inserter and not the low-status "punk", or insertee.) Luis begged to come back into the program, agreeing to talk about his problems. So, at the next community meeting I passed along his request, and the community voted him back in. Luis's behavior did not change, however. He revealed nothing. I took Luis aside and privately said to him, "Look, Luis, you promised to talk about things."

"[Sigh] How could you be so dumb? How could I talk about that kind of stuff when I'm both a leader of the Mexican Mafia and a high status inmate? Don't you know enough about cons by now to know that my position would be destroyed if I ever implied anything of that sort?"

"Well, what shall we do then?"

Luis couldn't come up with any answers.

Two intervening events occurred. Other prisoners saw Luis kissing a prisoner from another unit. (Mingling with prisoners from other units was not permitted.) A fellow prisoner had also observed him using burnt cork to enhance the attractiveness of his eyes. Consequently, at the next community meeting someone hooted, in a hardly sensitive manner, "Well, guess who's the faggot around here?" Luis immediately decompensated and became violent, assuming that I had betrayed him. Of course, I had not. Having become violent and uncontrollable, Luis had to be removed from the unit and was remanded to the maximum security Folsom State Penitentiary.

Many months later, I was in my small apartment alone in a not-very-good neighborhood, feeling quite depressed about my personal life. (I had been recently divorced, and my former wife and children were living in the lovely, big old house.) An elderly Caucasian gentleman knocked at my door asking to use the phone to call a cab. I said, "No, you can't come in; however, I'd be glad to call a taxi for you, give the driver directions, and tell you their estimate of how long it will take for the cab to get here." I closed the door, but did not lock it. A burly, young Mexican-American brandishing a large knife burst in announcing that he had just gotten out of Folsom and that Luis, as leader of the Mexican Mafia, had sent him to kill me. He apprised me of the facts that not only had he killed a number of people previously but also he enjoyed the act of killing as well as the sight of blood. I tried futilely to grab his arm; he hurled me across the room. Obviously, I could not overpower him physically. The only way in which I could possibly overcome him would be through wit and intellect. I was not stronger, but I was smarter. I would have to be totally unemotional, totally "left-brained". I was essentially a dead man; I had nothing to lose.

My intended assassin told me to lie down on the bed, informing me that he knew where my jugular vein and carotid artery were and that he would slice them open. Before I lay down, I told him that I was interested in the physiology of emotion and that I first wanted to check my pulse. He looked at me rather oddly as I counted my pulse, which was 80—my normal rate. I felt absolutely calm and rational. I figured that my only hope was to do the unexpected. (I presumed that he might expect me to plead or beg for my life.) As I lay on the bed and he teasingly began scratching at my neck with the knife, I said loudly and strongly, *[here the delicate reader should skip ahead because I am going to use some pretty rough language]* "Hey punk, how does it feel to get fucked in the ass, punk? [And since different ethnic groups do not generally get along with one another in prison] I bet you like a black cock, don't you punk, because it's bigger [playing into a prevalent myth, having no objective data on the subject]. How does it feel to have a thick black cock up your ass punk?"

"You're calling me a punk?!"

Deciding that the Ethics Committee of the American Psychiatric Association would permit my betrayal of confidence at this point, I queried, "Why are you here?"

"I already told you, because Luis sent me here to kill you."

"I know that, but *why* did Luis send you to kill me?"

"I don't know."

"Well, I'm going to tell you the absolute honest-to-God truth, and you can believe me or not." I told him the story.

"Gee, Doc, I didn't know Luis was a punk. I'm sorry, Doc; I would never have scared you and done this if I realized he was a punk." With that, he left quickly and quietly, taking nothing.

The instant he left, my heart began pounding furiously. I took my pulse again; it was 180. I was drenched in sweat and trembling. (The adaptive *postponement* of both psychological and physiological reactions to imminent danger that allowed rational, nonemotional coping was a remarkable phenomenon. My own "experiment" in mind-body unity, in which there was neither fear nor sympathetic nervous system reaction during intellectual coping, made me all the more convinced that my earlier basic premises in PNI were correct.) I called my best friend, a very muscular, former defensive lineman who had played on winning teams in the Sugar Bowl and Cotton Bowl. I told him to come over to my place quickly and to tell his wife that he would not return that evening but would call from my house to explain why. I wanted to be protected by the largest person I knew. I remained fearful and paranoid for about a year afterward, always on the lookout for trouble. I had a large variety of locks installed on my door. Did I call the police? No. Confident in my reputation for making a genuine effort to help our clients succeed in society, I called a former member of the Mexican Mafia who had completed our program and told him what happened. He immediately offered, "I'll get Luis killed for you."

"No. I'd like you to take care of the matter without killing Luis, but I don't want to get killed. I'm scared to death. He could send someone else after me. You take care of it without killing him and then tell me how you've done so."

A few months later he called me. We met, and he explained that the Mexican Mafia had sent one of its group members to Folsom, pretending that he could only speak Spanish and claiming to be a cousin of Luis's visiting from Mexico. The "relative" had conned his way into getting a single visit (not being on the visitor list) with Luis, to whom he issued the threat: "If anything violent happens to Solomon, you'll be dead in prison the next day." It must have worked. I'm still alive.

Our Model Treatment Program reduced recidivism within the year after release from over 90% to about 50%, but we did not have long term follow-up statistics, which I presume would reflect higher recidivism. Clearly, the program was much too brief, and I came away with the following conclusions in dealing with criminal offenders. First time offenders should not get probation. They should be given short sentences in correctional settings with other first offenders, preventing exposure to the crime-inducing ways of hard-core criminals. Probably 50% of first offenders (the "healthier") would learn from *experience* that one does not get away with crime. This practice would be quite inexpensive. Why treat those who do not need treatment? Overcrowded courts lead to too many lenient plea-bargain deals that actually reinforce criminal behaviors.

For those who become second offenders, I would offer (not require) an intensive treatment program similar to the one that we had attempted—but for much longer duration, probably three years. In order to participate in such a treatment program, however, the prisoner would need to demonstrate motivation *behaviorally*, as well as verbally, by giving up free time and agreeing to incarceration for a longer period of time. In other words, "We'll try to help you have a productive life in society if you're willing to invest some additional time in the joint to accomplish that." I would also provide vocational training and substance abuse treatment because one who cannot work or give up an addiction is far more likely to revert to crime. Only for a third offense after treatment would I be amenable to a "three strikes and you're out" approach (for serious offenses only). I strongly feel that this policy is unfair to apply without first providing an opportunity for rehabilitation.

Youngsters in their early teens who get in serious trouble have the best prospects for rehabilitation because they are old enough to take responsibility for their actions but not so old as to be set in their ways. These juvenile offenders need to be provided with suitable identification figures, attention, care, training, and probably foster homes with continued supervision and help. "Smart ass" late adolescent and early adult prisoners are the most difficult group with which to work.

Effective means of preventing violence remain elusive. They would require eradicating or reducing the factors common to the backgrounds of violent offenders: blatant inconsistencies in parental behavior; violence in the home, to which the child is either witness or victim; gross lack of affection, including lack of basic positive regard for the child; and actual loss of or virtually complete separation from one or both parents. Stated differently, prevention would entail promoting consistent, fair, and affectionate childrearing. This level of prevention is called primary prevention. Early identification of and treatment for children at risk of antisocial behavior and substance abuse, as a means of curbing later violent offenses, constitutes secondary prevention. Forewarnings of potential for later destructive behavior include: a history of actual incidents of violent and destructive behavior; poorly controlled anger and excessive response to minor frustrations or, conversely, marked overcontrol and the inability to express any resentment; repeated behavioral problems in the classroom; and parental neglect or abuse perpetrated upon the child. Targeting such children, however, may create self-fulfilling prophecies, since children often live up to their inevitable labels. Therefore, all people, especially children, need be taught to view anger as a signal to identify a problem and enlist appropriate coping responses, such as the verbal expression of feelings or the discharging of emotion through other activities such as sports and nonviolent protest.

Prisons are full of opportunities for destructive and manipulative behavior; relationships are based upon power and exploitation. The psychopath does not trust. It is hard to find anyone trustworthy in a prison, either staff member or inmate. The psychopath acts out of expediency and narrow self-interest. There are few opportunities for long-term, goal-directed behavior or for behaving in terms of the good of the group in prison. The psychopath has often been a victim of brutality and abuse; in prison, he still may be, at the hands of his keepers. In childhood, parents and others did not spontaneously meet his needs out of understanding and concern. Needs are hardly so met in prison.

The correctional system and its inmate subculture, replete with con bosses, is based on coercion, fear, and power. Slyness and deceit are likely to pay off. Sexuality is expressed in the service of dominance, exploitation, and tension relief rather than in terms of appropriate affectionate bonds. Relationships are generally superficial and lacking in deep emotionality. One's bad and worthless self-concept is reinforced. It is hard to find any suitable role models. The acquisition of adaptive and coping skills, both vocational and psychological, is neglected. The criminal is usually ignorant and untrained. Prisons often offer some educational opportunities, but vocational training is rare. Idle time is not only useless but also destructive. Surely more than TV sets and weight rooms should be provided. "Doing time" is thus reduced to living in the moment. It seems that society has designed a system that effectively reinforces criminal behavior. A convict writes, "The correctional system could be compared to a patient entering a hospital for an appendectomy and coming out with a terminal case of cancer." Karl Menninger, of the renowned multigenerational family of prominent psychiatrists, stated, "*I suspect that all crimes committed by all the jailed criminals do not equal in total the social damage of the crimes committed against them.*"

The following passage on the rehabilitation of criminals comes from the "Statement of Twenty-Two Principles" drawn up at the first meeting of the American Correctional Association in *1870*:

"Reformation, not vindictive suffering, should be the purpose of the penal treatment of prisoners. The prisoner should be made to realize that his destiny is in his own hands. Prison discipline should be such as to gain the will of the prisoner and conserve his self-respect. The aim of the prison should be to make industrious free men rather than orderly and obedient prisoners."

Certainly, the mental health professional, or any staff person interfacing with prison inmates for that matter, should be committed to the view that human behavior can be modified, that human beings have a natural tendency toward adaptation and maturation. More important than any specific treatment technique or administrative policy is an atmosphere of general optimism, helpfulness, empathy, and concern combined with programmatic dedication to structure, mutual respect, and individual responsibility for behavior. Meaningful involvement with other individuals develops self-worth, from which follows the capacity for empathy, which in turn prevents the victimization of others. Even late, some rehabilitation or "tertiary prevention" may be possible.

It is ludicrous to expect that a prisoner can abruptly make the transition from a maximum security setting to complete freedom; therefore, opportunity must be provided for trial and error, while offering protection to the inmate and community. Ideally, soon-to-be-released offenders should be housed in relatively small and secure local facilities, such as modified county jails, that provide training, probationary supervision, work furlough programs, and halfway houses. In order to be accepted by the community, such a system must be compatible with existing organizational structures: courts, probation departments, law enforcement agencies, and mental health departments. An alien program patched onto the criminal justice system would soon be rejected like a graft from a nonmatched donor.

Joe was a criminal in his early 30s who spent roughly half his life in various penal institutions. As a graduate of the Model Treatment

Program in Fresno County, he spoke publicly of how his life was essentially shaped by his experiences in those institutions. Joe received his initiation into a life of crime when he was sent to a reformatory in California at the age of 14. In the reformatory, Joe swiftly discovered what he had to do to survive:

"I had to live . . . according to the cons' code . . . I knew that I had to exist in that fuckin' environment. I was used. I used to do things for them that they themselves wouldn't do, such as jump on the . . . counselor in the dormitory, jump on people that were outside of the cliques to prove my manhood which I didn't want to [do] . . . When I was in school there were times when I couldn't even stand being around my own people 'cause I hated some of the things that they were doing, so I'd find a reason to get away from them. Go to the restroom or do extra work or something."

A few years later at Tracy State Penitentiary, he began adopting the "convict code" as a way of life because the stakes were even higher; prison was no longer just about survival, it was about power and acceptance:

"I went to Tracy . . . it's pretty heavy. I was one of the younger dudes there. There was a lot of lifers there then . . . Went there for assault and stealing a car I think it was. Didn't even go to school . . . take vocational training. . . . because I was part of a clique that . . . didn't want to deal with the system. Didn't want to deal with anything outside of ourselves other than to get high and run things in the penitentiary as far as poker games and pressuring people for their commissary, selling punks and all that shit . . . I was already boxing then . . . featherweight champion there, so I had a lot of prestige amongst the cons there. I was well liked, a lot of influence amongst them, especially because of the clique that I belonged to. Powerfullest one there. So I had everything going for myself as far as being involved in all the wheeling and dealing . . . I wanted to do something for myself but like I said is I just couldn't. The forces were so strong. They were holding me back. Convict code. I was too deep off in it . . . He [the psychiatrist] tried to give me some kind of ideas as to how I can get out from being part of the clique, but I just couldn't because I knew that if I got out the consequences was that I was gonna have to pick up a knife and to kill somebody or be killed."

Joe found the correctional staff to be sadistic, using torture as the mode of discipline, which only served to breed hatred:

"They used to put me in the cooler [solitary confinement]. I couldn't stand it. I used to holler. Fuck, I thought I was going crazy . . . I wanted to kill myself. And I just started gettin' really a lot of hatred in me. And all I was thinkin' about was I'm gonna kill the son-of-a-bitch. I'm gonna kill somebody. I'm gonna kill somebody. I'm gonna get even. I'm gonna get even. Cause they had no right to do that to me . . . they used their own fuckin' methods of trying to correct me, makin' me behave, by usin' damn clubs and gas, puttin' me in the damn ice box, in the cooler and giving me RD, which was just like a meatloaf type of frozen food. That once a day and in the evenings, you know, they come over there and give me a medicine cup of water. I'd starve, fuckin'-A just starve . . . Everytime I'd come out of the damn hole [solitary confinement] man, they'd just be waiting, five, six, seven of them, and they'd ask me how I felt, if I was all right, and I says, 'Yeah.' That hatred was in my heart, and they can see it in my eyes and right away they start bouncing me off the damn walls again because as far as they was concerned I wasn't even corrected. And you know what? . . . I'm not bullshittin'. If I had a knife in my hand then—any kind of a weapon—believe me, I'd have killed somebody. Anyway, eventually they let me go back on the damn yard. I was always scheming a way to get back at these fools."

The prisoners were stripped of rights and helpless to all the meaningless brutality:

"One fuckin' day they call me over, and they says, 'Look, this is what we're gonna do to you if you don't straighten out,' and they killed a guy right in front of my eyes. They put his damn head on the damn bars and they just beat him to dead like if it was nothing. And they'd laugh. And the guy that killed him stood about six-foot three-and-a-half, weighed about 220 pounds. And I know his damn name, too. I was right there when he killed him. But it just so happens, you know what, that I was a damn convict, and I didn't have no fuckin' say so and they would never believe me in fuckin' court because of my fuckin'-minded behavior and because of the fuckin' psychotic jacket [classification] that they hung on me and all that book shit. And they wanted to keep me buried . . . because of the crowd that I hung around with. I was the only witness there. All of them were officers. I don't know how many other times they beat people like that."

When psychotherapy groups were available, they were a joke:

"In Soledad [State Penitentiary] I wanted to do somethin' for myself as far as education, and them counseling groups they got there ain't nothing. You sit down and talk about French toast, how poor the chow is, the TV's fucked up, the man's pickin' on me, how come we can't have this, the showers are fucked up, how come we can't have no more recreation activities, how come the visits are like this, all just a bunch of bullshit. They weren't really dealing with nothing. I wanna start dealing with something about my personal hangups, but I couldn't because there were 50-80 men in each community group, and they were supposed to be talkin' about problems that got people involved in crime and penitentiaries. And they're talkin' about all this other bullshit that didn't pertain nothin' about gettin' oneself together. So they're talkin' about how to better things in the penitentiary, so they can stay there, so they can pacify them. Well, I don't want to talk about that. So I sit there and stand mute. Didn't say a damn fuckin' thing. Nothing. Well, I did get involved by myself in AA [Alcoholics Anonymous] because while it was open anybody could go in there. I'd just sit there and drink coffee, hear some of the guys. I wanted to get up and talk about my experience, my life and everything, my problems, but I couldn't because people that I associated with were there. I was afraid of what they would think."

When he got to Folsom State Penitentiary, the other state penitentiaries looked lightweight by comparison:

"I went to Folsom because the staff feared me because of the clique that I was involved in, even though we weren't doin' really anything drastic, violent. I was one of the youngest dudes there . . . I was scared well because it was hard core people that are there 15, 20, 25, 30, and 35 fuckin' years . . . I couldn't identify with all the people there, but I had to . . . So I started pickin' up that old con bullshit again and gettin' into hassles, gambling, running fuckin' games, booze, fuckin' with punks. Well I got my ass beaten there . . . by some sadistic professional people. 'Cause right there they'd tell you, 'You know what? This is Folsom. We have our own rules around here, and we're gonna deal with you. We don't give a shit where you've been, how old you are, what color you are,' and then he handcuffs you and not one or two or three whip on you. Five, six, and seven, they take turns. And after you're knocked out, they wake you up and come back. You think you're dead, or you wanna die if you're not dead. If the doctor comes down there and sees you aren't okay, and he patches you up, you know, and he leaves. And then after you're together again, you know what, they come in there and whip the shit out of you again . . . People didn't even have it coming."

The ultimate hell was Minnesota State Penitentiary:

"The first thing I encountered was the silent treatment. The canes. The most awful sadistic son-of-a-bitches that I ever met, the staff there . . . I was the only Chicano in that damn penitentiary. I was doin' 20 years. I had 13 years, 11 months, 27 days . . . before I'd even be considered for parole. How in the hell was I gonna live, man, with the silent treatment, canes, watchin' them people usin' canes on them poor dudes, no yard, shower once a week, food messed up, no TV; they never saw a TV there, not even the radio? I read about such things. I couldn't believe it. Then they had twine shop, slave shop making twine. It's the only thing they had. They had a couple of other little things, machine shop, a foundry, making farm machinery for farmers out there . . . They had no ethnic groups, no course of studies; they had no education for nobody; they had no vocational training; they had no group counseling, no therapeutic sessions; they had one psychologist and all he done was just kick back and done board reports and that's it. And I had one fuckin' counselor didn't do one fuckin' thing but come in there and get high on grass and that was it and bullshit."

There, all efforts on the part of prisoners to take nonviolent initiative were met with extreme violence:

"So because I was a Chicano dude and I was following with some good people and I had influence, done time in Folsom, San Quentin, Soledad, they respected me. And then the grapevine, they got some good feedback on me . . . We all got together in . . . the block that I was livin' in and we just decided work stoppage till we got some answers, till we started gettin' some programs in there; education was one of the main concerns and better visits, better chow. Damn warden come over there and broke the damn window and he says, 'You have three minutes to clear the damn hallway up. You don't want us, but we're comin' in.' And they had riot guns, they had machine guns, they had 45 caliber pistols, they had huntin' rifles and shotguns and I don't know what else. And we all's a peaceful demonstration. He said, 'You got three minutes.' No sooner than he said that, when he start firing away. Three dudes died, 11 were wounded. . . . Even the doctors couldn't believe it. I was one of the leaders . . . They were out to kill me and some other . . . dudes . . . They locked everybody up. They took 47 of us, 46 were Indians, I was the only Chicano. They didn't touch any other person. They took us up to the education department. They said they want to talk to us. They sat us all down, they put chairs in front of us, and they was in front of us. And the fuckin' fools they came in there and just popped gas and started swinging clubs, and behind them there was officers with weapons. What the fuck for? . . . See we let 'em beat on us, but I didn't. There was two of us that didn't. I ended up in the damn hospital. The other guy ended up in the hospital in the university on the streets. After I got out of the damn hospital they came to threaten me at the hospital that if I was going to testify that I would never see the streets. They would show me what they meant . . . As far as I was concerned I was decided to . . . So they put me in the hole for awhile. They didn't fuck with me in the hole. I didn't have nothin' to read, didn't have no clothes, didn't have no mattress, had to sleep on the damn cold floor. All this time that I was gettin' visits, Mona used to come over. I wanted to love her. I wanted to give her my heart. I couldn't. I couldn't because I was too fuckin' deep off in this fuckin' shit and they were tryin' to make a mother fuckin' animal out of me. They really were."

The transition from prison to civilian life proved too much to bear:

"I didn't wanna leave 'cause I wasn't ready for the streets even though I had been involved in education, trying to get myself together. There were still other hangups that I had within myself as far as fear, as far as whether I should go back into crime, or get involved in a militant bag on the violence side of it and start bombin' these prisons and everything you know. Or get involved on the social side . . . and get involved in tryin' to come into these prisons and everything and helpin' people out . . . So I contacted some people that were just starting to build a halfway rehab house, some chapter of Synanon near Minneapolis. I talked to 'em and told 'em what my problems was. As far as I was concerned I wasn't ready . . . I says,' . . . I'm willin' to give . . . everything up . . . just to go over there at your rehab house and get my shit together, get me strong enough so I can go out there and relate to people man. Right now I feel violent, I feel that I just wanna destroy everything, the system and everything. I know there's better ways, there's other avenues to take, I says, but right now you know I'm not ready.' . . . I was there a month and a half. Got too heavy for me. Stripped me of all my identity. . . . Started tryin' to deal with myself and at the same time I was dealing with problems outside of myself—my wife, rent, hospital bills, car payments, insurance, things of that nature. And then I was gettin' feedback from people that I knew in the streets, 'Well, come on now, we have a [drug] bag waiting for you. We want you to run for us. You know there's money available for you.' Things of that nature. Back in fuckin' crime . . . So anyway I was starting to fuck around with drugs again. Too confused. Just couldn't deal with it, deal with my problems. Too confused."

Back at Folsom State Penitentiary, Joe finally feigned psychosis as a last resort, only to encounter atrocities of an entirely different nature in the psych unit:

"I said, 'Fuck it, I'm gonna just transfer on out.' To transfer on outs I gotta play a psych role. That was the only way and you gotta play a hell of a good psych role. So I played a psych role that I was paranoid. So I convinced the doctor pretty good, 'Do you want me to put you on medication?' I says, 'No, I don't want to deal with it that way. That'll just corrupt the issue, problems.' . . . They had a psych unit where they . . . medicate them dudes down there, got 'em crawlin' on their hands and knees like they were animals instead of really dealing with them as if they were people with problems. And they call themselves concerned, qualified professional people to deal with people that have problems . . . They ain't qualified. I came there. They were afraid because they couldn't get me on medication. They tried to force me. Well I was stupid. For about two weeks, I was on medication, Valiums® and some kind of sleepers. I can't remember the names, some red, looks like jelly beans, some kind of liquid, Darvons® . . . Well out there, I was slick; I thought I was gonna get high. They didn't do a fuckin' thing but make me sick. I couldn't even take care of myself, couldn't even shave, couldn't even clothe myself right, and I like to take care of myself. I like to get clean. I couldn't even walk. I couldn't even talk to people. Saliva comin' out of my mouth man when I eat, messin' like spit all over my food . . . Custody ain't supposed to run nothing other than disciplinary and security. That is all. The hospital's supposed to be run by the doctors, the psychiatric staff. The psychiatrists, they're easily boss there, and yet custody was the one that pulls the guy out of the cell and says, 'Come here.' . . . They yank him out, they whip on him, and they take him over and they says, 'Give this man medication.' The NTA [psychiatric orderly] says 'What happened?' 'This man jumped on one of the officers and this man is very violent so give him a shot of Thorazine® or Prolixin®, or whatever.' And then they strip the guy and put him in what they call a P cell, a psychotic cell. Nothing in there but a piece of slab . . . I'm tryin' to help some of these guys get away from the medication and tell staff, 'Fuck you, I don't want this guy to be on medication no more.' 'Well who are you?' . . . I say, 'Hey, I'm just living with this guy here you know in this institution, this guy that's been on medication. You people . . . just got him on medications just to keep him out of your face. You know what? You're not helpin' this guy, you're destroyin' him, you're burnin' him out . . . and that's not right.' . . .

Sayin' that they're helpin' him. Well that's bullshit. They got the guy. Everytime that he wakes up, they give him a shot to knock him out. The poor guy wakes up, he can't even talk. They ask him, 'How do you feel there, uh, John?' 'UhuhUhuh.' They give him another shot and knock him out. I seen it with my own eyes. I know it happened to me, too, 'cause I was out for three fuckin' days. Three days."

While running the Model Treatment Program in Fresno, I was called as a psychiatric expert witness in several highly publicized, controversial criminal cases. (In criminal forensics, the psychiatrist informs the hiring attorney's client that what he or she says will be revealed in totality to and be used at the sole discretion of the attorney: "attorney's privilege", rather than "patient's privilege" regarding confidentiality). These psychiatric examinations encourage scrutiny of the criminal justice system and what it means to have a "fair trial". These cases will illustrate the complexity of the issues. (The O.J. Simpson trial, at which there was no psychiatric testimony, will hopefully lead to more such scrutiny about the issue of fairness.)

Defendant: Dan White
Male, Caucasian
Late 30s, Married
Charge: First degree murder with special circumstances: shooting to
    death San Francisco Mayor George Moscone and Supervisor
    Harvey Milk, the first openly gay supervisor in San Francisco
Verdict: Guilty of voluntary manslaughter

The Dan White case was among the most tragic and misunderstood cases I ever encountered. Distortion of facts by the media was appalling in this highly politicized case. Mayor George Moscone and Supervisor Harvey Milk were highly respected—even beloved—by the San Francisco community. As its first avowedly gay supervisor, Harvey Milk was a rightful hero to the City's large and politically conscious gay community. From this case I learned the hazards of pretrial media coverage and the importance of nonprejudgment, since Dan was so different than I had expected him to be. (About 70% of the time, my assessments do not support the position of the attorneys who have called me; therefore, although I have done a good number of examinations, I have been called to testify relatively infrequently.) There were scores of psychiatrists and psychologists who sounded off about Dan's presumed hypermasculinity, homophobia, latent homosexuality, and paranoia. He was none of those things. On the surface, it seemed apparent that Dan had entered City Hall, avoiding the metal detector, with a loaded gun in order to kill the Mayor and probably the Supervisor as well. As the case evolved, there was no evidence for premeditation. The defense, which was not making a case for insanity but for diminished (mental) capacity to form specific intent, was continually held up for ridicule as the "Twinkie defense".

Dan was very fond of both his parents. His father was a proud member of the Irish community in San Francisco, happily serving as both policeman and fireman. Following in his father's footsteps, Dan served as a policeman in San Francisco. He was a highly religious man whose strong sense of principles were of the "black and white" variety, not allowing for many "shades of gray". His Irish Catholic background and strict upbringing made him highly self-critical and prone to feelings of inadequacy, depression, and guilt when he fell short of his own high expectations. For instance, after having observed a fellow policeman beating a shackled prisoner, he turned in the officer for brutality. (It is an unwritten rule that you don't "rat" on another policeman.) Dan's betrayal made him *persona non grata* to his colleagues, and he was made to feel so uncomfortable that he left the police force. Far happier as a fireman, Dan came to feel that he could do some good as a politician, for he could never deal with politics as the art of compromise. Popularity within his blue collar community led to his election to the City and County (combined in San Francisco) Board of Supervisors. After winning the election, however, it was decided that his position as a city fireman represented a potential conflict of interest for his supervisorial responsibilities. He was forced to give up being a fireman. Supervisors' salaries were only about $1,000 per month; so, in order to make ends meet, his pregnant wife had to run a hot dog stand for tourists visiting Pier 39 near Fisherman's Wharf. (Dan's wife was an absolutely lovely, devoted woman who married Dan, her first and only intimate partner, in her mid-30s).

There was ample evidence that Dan was not the anti-gay, right-wing bigot that the gay community viewed him to be. One of his varsity baseball team buddies from St. Ignatius High School (a boys' parochial secondary school in San Francisco) made it to the major leagues, during which time it became known to the public (and Dan) that he was gay. Dan subsequently led a campaign to have his friend reinstated onto the major league team on the basis that his sexual preference had nothing to do with his athletic capabilities. Further-more, although Dan's political views leaned toward the right, the only two supervisors he respected were liberals Dianne Feinstein, now Senator Feinstein, and Harvey Milk, whom he regarded as hav-ing integrity in that they could not be bought off with money. This integrity was particularly impressive in Harvey's case, as he was a man of little means. Despite his largely blue collar constituency, Dan accompanied Harvey to a gay rights rally and to a lesbian gathering. Harvey's honesty and underdog status had made Dan an admirer. During this period, Dan cast the deciding vote for Dianne to become Chair of the Board of Supervisors. In an act of gratitude, she asked what she could do for him. He replied, "Make Harvey Chairman of the Transportation Committee." Dan knew that Harvey had wanted the chairmanship and would do justice to the role in spite of their differences in political viewpoint. Nevertheless, Dianne would not appoint Harvey because of his refusal to support her otherwise unani-mous election.

Counter to Dan's apparent strength, he suffered from atypically brief bouts of severe clinical depression (to psychotic degree, in my opinion), lasting from days to a couple of weeks at a time. During these periods, he would break from his fitness and health food rou-tine, closing himself up in his bedroom to watch television, read, and eat junk food. He would withdraw and "hate myself and everyone else". (One of the three defense psychiatrists, Martin Blinder, happened to mention the name "Twinkies" along with a casual theory, which I considered to be weak, that the gorging may have contributed to a blood sugar imbalance, possibly affecting his thinking—hence, the term "Twinkie defense".) Major depressive disorder has two predominant vegetative (bodily) symptoms: sleep disturbance (usually insomnia and early morning awakening but sometimes hypersomnia, or sleeping much of the time—which Dan did) and appetite disturbance (usually anorexia, or lack of appetite, but sometimes hyperphagia, or gorging—which Dan also did). Another symptom is loss of libido, which Dan experienced when he was depressed. Realizing that these symptoms would eventually subside, Dan merely withdrew during his periods of depression and never sought treatment.

In the face of mounting financial pressures because of the sacrifice of his job as a fireman and a baby on the way, Dan became particularly incensed that he had been required to give up the joy and security of his job to prevent a conflict of interest while he was observing other supervisors acquiring thousands of dollars from developers by granting building permits, and this payoff was not viewed as a conflict of interest. As it became increasingly difficult to make ends meet, he began suffering from unrelenting depression and, therefore, resigned as a supervisor. Much relieved, Dan spent the summer at lovely Lake Tahoe in the Sierra Mountains with his wife and newborn child, feeling well and planning to return to the fire department. The respite was brief, however. Depression returned with a vengeance when he was made to feel that he had let down his constituents, who were concerned that the Mayor would appoint a liberal to take the vacant seat, altering the political balance of the board. Obligingly, he consulted the Mayor about the possibility of reinstatement, to which the Mayor responded affirmatively. Although they had disagreed on politics, the Mayor liked and respected Dan as a person. Nonetheless, responding to tremendous political pressure from his liberal supporters, the Mayor reneged on his agreement with Dan. Making matters worse, when Dan was in the City Attorney's office attempting to get a ruling on the legality of his reappointment, he

overheard a telephone conversation in which Harvey Milk was lobbying for the rejection of his request in favor of placing another liberal on the board. Even Harvey was not above realpolitik.

All but two of the supervisors routinely carried guns in light of
recurring death threats. (Once, a gun had come in handy to display
when Dan was threatened with assault on a bus.) In Dan's trial, Dianne
Feinstein admitted that she had carried a gun in her purse at almost
all times and had taken the Police Academy course in pistol shooting.
The supervisors would routinely walk around the metal detector or
enter the building by the basement window in order to avoid detec-
tion. Dan had not actually intended to go to City Hall the morning of
the killings. It was only after his aide had called and asked him to
assist her and some supporters in getting to see the Mayor that, after
an initial refusal, he reluctantly agreed to go. Although he clearly
bore some resentment toward the Mayor, Dan's conscious intent as he
entered the building on the day of the murder was to beg for reappointment. Albeit cordially, the Mayor refused to do so, at which
moment Dan fired at him five times, killing him. Three to five minutes later, after reloading his revolver, Dan walked over to Harvey
Milk's office across the hall and killed him. The reloading of the
revolver appeared to be evidence of premeditation for killing the Supervisor. Dan explained, however, that at the Police Academy he had
been trained always to reload after shooting, and I believed him. I
asked him why he went to see Harvey. He said that he had intended
to beg Harvey to intervene on his behalf to change the Mayor's mind
about his being reappointed (after he had already shot the Mayor five
times, hardly rational!) Dan thoroughly denied any conscious prior
intent to kill either the Mayor or Harvey Milk:

"Everything I believed in was being crushed. There was no human factor. Whatever happened to me, my family did not matter. I felt
totally helpless. I just shot him (the Mayor) . . . Living one's life
trying to do the right thing led to this."

Was he legally insane? (Dan was at the very least in the same
mental state when he shot Harvey as he was when he shot the Mayor.)
I had taken the conservative position that he was legally sane. I also

felt, however, that there was absolutely no evidence of premeditation; his action was essentially instantaneous with both the Mayor and Harvey. (Don Lunde, a forensic psychiatrist for whom I have much regard, and who is a friend as well, came up with an assessment virtually identical to mine.) Dan stated that he had killed Harvey because he thought he had a seen a smirk on his face. The issue of malice was more questionable since Dan bore some resentment toward the Mayor and Harvey. I, therefore, expected him to be convicted of second-degree murder. I was surprised by the verdict of voluntary manslaughter.

Dan White falls in the category of "overcontrolled" killers. Although he had become a good fighter in self-defense, he had had great difficulty expressing anger, however appropriate. When I asked, "Why didn't you tell the Mayor off and call him a two-timing son-of-a-bitch for reneging on his promise to reappoint you?" Dan replied something to the effect, "That would have been extremely discourteous." Psychiatrist Emanuel Tanay seemed to be talking about Dan when he described the "aggressophobic personality", one capable of committing homicide "out of character". Such individuals are rigid, moralistic, and highly conflicted about their own aggressive strivings. They have an overdeveloped "internal parent" that is demanding, cruel, and unpredictable in approval—very much like the parents they had as children. The aggressophobe shows an inability to express aggression on all levels. Absence of aggressive fantasies is also part of the package. Their repressed aggressions are, therefore, projected upon others. The aggressophobe appears reserved and pleasant in contrast to the "undercontrolled" personality who attracts conflict by behaving "with a chip on the shoulder". I told the court that because of Dan's extremely strong conscience, he would inevitably feel a great deal of guilt and remorse about his actions (which most people did not believe that he felt). I anticipated that were he not significantly punished, he would ultimately punish himself. Likewise, were he not treated for depression while incarcerated, he would be suicidal.

Years later, after Dan's release from prison, a San Francisco newspaper headline read, "A Psychiatrist's Prediction Comes True". Dan had killed himself. I had advised against his return to San Francisco, encouraging him to follow his longtime dream of living in Ireland. He had returned, nonetheless, because of his family and his wife's job. Mrs. White had become pregnant again as the result of a conjugal visit in prison. Their second child had been born with Down's syndrome, and his wife, then in her 40s, was still struggling to support their children.

My own mother was furious at me for testifying in Dan White's defense. Mayor Moscone had been a friend of hers, having dropped her off at home after a party only a few nights prior to his death. "How could you defend my friend's killer?," she snapped. I had been surprised by my own findings; I had not anticipated serious psychopathology other than character disorder. Once that I had agreed to examine Dan, I felt a moral responsibility to state my opinion, even if it offended the gay community or my mother. I did in fact offend the gay community, as evidenced by a number of death threats that came my way. Ridiculously, some accused me of being homophobic, but at that time I felt unable to defend myself. (Despite my openness later during my time with the Biopsychosocial AIDS Project at UCSF, I still had difficulty with some who recalled my involvement in the Dan White case.) I have always been supportive of memorial programs in honor of Harvey Milk. In many ways he was a true hero, even if his tragic death was not directly related to being gay. I was only upset with the portrayal of Dan White as a hideous, anti-gay villain, rather than as the basically decent but extremely emotionally troubled man that he was—one who perpetrated an awful crime during an episode of irrationality for which he ultimately paid the price of death. Gay people, like other minorities, are not immune from bias.

Defendant: Edmund Kemper
Male, Caucasian
24 years old, Single
Charge: First degree murder with special circumstances: serial kill-
   ing of eight young coeds
Verdict: Guilty of first degree murder

Edmund Kemper was a highly intelligent and physically impos-
ing man of six-feet nine-inches and 280 pounds, the middle of three
children from a broken family. After his parents separated, Edmund
almost never saw his father, which embittered him toward his mother,
who had sabotaged contact with his father. From Edmund's perspective, his mother's role as a single parent consisted solely of castigation
and ridicule. The enormous antipathy that he developed toward his
mother gradually generalized to other women. As a boy, Edmund
indulged in fantasies of killing women, his mother in particular. Due
to his sense of sexual and social inadequacy, he also fantasized making
love to corpses. He believed a living woman would make fun of his
small penis (whether actually small or only in relation to his huge
body, I have no idea). Edmund was fascinated with weapons and
execution, playacting his own suffocation in a gas chamber and chop-
ping up neighborhood cats in his spare time. He was never actually
caught for the cat killings, having developed an uncanny ability to lie.
(The police didn't even believe his confession, years later, until he was
able to produce bodies.)

At the age of 13, Edmund ran away from home, but his attempt
to live with his father met with rejection. Consequently, against his
will, his mother sent him to live with his grandparents on their se-
cluded ranch. There, Edmund's murder history began at age 15, less
than a year after he moved in with his grandparents, when he shot
and then repeatedly stabbed his grandmother to death. He claimed
that she was a vicious, hostile woman (with whom his mother evidently had identified). According to what Edmund told me, he then

shot his grandfather, the only male he ever killed, in order to spare him being a lonely widower. (I believe that he killed his grandfather mainly to cover up the murder of his grandmother.) After the first double homicide, he phoned his mother and waited for the authorities to take him away.

Edmund was found not guilty by reason of insanity and was sent, even as a teenager, to Atascadero. There he worked in the psychology laboratory where he was able, with his brilliant mind, to memorize normal responses to standard psychological tests, including the projective Rorschach and Thematic Apperception Tests. (Although some of Edmund's test results during this time showed unstability, impulsivity, and general distress, they ultimately proved to be diagnostically useless.) In a routine follow-up visit after his release at age 21, the examining psychiatrist concluded that the only danger Edmund might pose to society would be hitting somebody while speeding on his motorcycle. The psychiatrist couldn't have been more bamboozled. (Edmund divulged to me later that, at the very moment he was being examined by the psychiatrist, in the trunk of his car was the body of one of his victims!) After discharge from Atascadero, Edmund was released to his mother by the parole board of the Youth Authority, which had not taken into account his psychiatric needs or his history of hostility toward his mother—a terrible mistake. The renewal of old dynamics with his mother, then on the administrative staff of the University of California, Santa Cruz, revived old fantasies and gave him access to a new type of surrogate victim: university coeds.

Edmund began by interviewing young women, mostly hitchhikers, for "victim suitability". Victims were either those he judged to be overprivileged on the one hand, or hippies, on the other. Strangely, he felt guilty about only one killing, a Japanese ballet dancer. Although she hadn't fit either of the two categories, he felt that through his line of questioning she had been catching on to the fact that he was the sought-after serial killer. I got the details of these killings in a voluntary narcoanalytic interview. Edmund did not want his victims to suffer; he merely wanted them dead. Except in two initial cases involving shooting and stabbing, he had perfected a very quick method of killing by snapping necks with his powerful arms to minimize suffering—essentially what happens during hanging. He then engaged in sexual activity with the corpses. Edmund revealed during this session that he then severed the legs of the bodies for freezing and subsequent cannibalism. [This interview (with the huge prisoner shackled to the bed and both a sheriff's deputy and a male nurse present) was one of two that I ever conducted during which I had to excuse myself for a few minutes in order not to disrupt "rapport" because I felt nauseated.] A new victim was "required" when the freezer was empty. The most bizarre aspect of this revolting tale, however, is the following. In light of his longtime wish to have been a policeman, Edmund frequented a Santa Cruz bar popular with off-duty police officers, whom he "befriended". They sometimes discussed the mystery of the serial killer. On occasion, Edmund invited them to his apartment for dinner and served "chicken casserole". In search of the serial killer, the policemen were actually eating the victims!

After killing eight young victims, Edmund finally killed his mother. First, he ripped out her larynx, so he could tell her things that he had been too afraid to say for fear of being yelled at. Then he decapitated the corpse. Next, he stuck her head on a pole, told her a lifetime's worth of built-up resentment, and smashed her face in with his fists. Following this catharsis, he left a cryptic note in his mother's apartment in hopes of a national manhunt. Alerts and bulletins not forthcoming, he uneventfully turned himself in, having to convince the police with several increasingly detailed phone messages that he was, indeed, the killer. One might speculate that, had he killed his mother first, all the other killings might not have been necessary.

Edmund Kemper's bizarre story led to further reassessment of what constitutes legal insanity. While utterly weird and virtually incomprehensible, his thinking and behavior were hard to classify in any standard diagnostic way. They were not characteristic of schizophrenia or manic-depressive (bipolar) psychosis (the two most common classes of mental illness). Although they did involve the paraphilic (obsessive, unusual sexual practices) perversion of necrophilia (literally "love of the dead"), they were not representative of classic sadism in that he neither tortured his victims nor engaged with *consenting* masochists. Edmund was found legally *sane*. It is difficult to generalize from such rare and bizarre cases. Such dangerous and likely untreatable persons probably need to be kept from society for a lifetime, but it is doubtful whether the usual prison setting would be appropriate. Edmund has been housed in a prison unit for mentally ill criminals.

Defendant: Leslie Van Houten
Female, Caucasian
Early 20s, Single
Charge: First degree murder: stabbing to death a woman (Mrs. La
  Bianca) during a Charles Manson "family" cult activity
Verdict: Guilty of first degree murder

Leslie Van Houten, one of the infamous Charles Manson women, was for all intents and purposes the opposite of Edmund Kemper. A basically nice and fairly normal young woman, Leslie had gotten caught up in an unforeseeably horrible situation (unlike most of the other Manson women who had actually sought out Manson for his cult-like activities). She had been introduced to Manson through her smooth and good-looking boyfriend, Charles "Tex" Watson. Although Manson had controlling sexual relationships with all the women in his following, the one person who could manipulate him was Tex, with whom Manson was captivated. Leslie accompanied Tex to the commune in the desert, which was allegedly concerned with ecology and opting out of a destructive society. Such missions were typical of communes in the '60s. Manson's group became isolated and engaged in increasingly bizarre behavior over time in conjunction with the use of vast amounts of LSD. Manson, whose baffling charisma compensated for his lack of education, would induce his followers into carrying out his dastardly plans while maintaining some personal distance from their actual execution. (Manson always refused psychiatric examination, but the extensive ranting evident throughout his correspondence with Leslie and Lynette "Squeaky" Fromme seemed quite psychotic to me.)

Leslie's initial trial led to a conviction of first degree murder and a sentence of life imprisonment; however, her trial had been marred by the disappearance of her lawyer. A replacement attorney assumed the case. Later, the original lawyer's body was discovered in the California desert. Although the cause of death was never precisely determined, the most benign explanation was that he, an avid hiker, had simply lost his way and died of dehydration and exhaustion. Of course, nefarious schemes have been speculated upon. After a number of appeals, spanning years, the California Supreme Court invalidated Leslie's conviction on the grounds that her second defense attorney had been unfamiliar with the case and, therefore, unprepared. She was actually out on bail for almost a year, causing no problems whatsoever. The second trial produced a hung jury. The third trial led to the actual conviction. (I testified in her second and third trials.)

Leslie had been a rather rebellious adolescent, but she did not come from a disturbed home; she had a relatively healthy relationship with all the members of her family. She showed no signs of significant psychopathology. Although initially continuing to correspond with Manson, Leslie seemed to recover from the effects of her cult indoctrination and to acquire some realistic perspective about what had transpired. There is a great deal of debate about brainwashing as a defense, even among those whom I most respect. For example, Jolly West and Margaret Thayler Singer, who both participated in the Patty Hearst case, believe in it; my friend Donald Lunde, who has written a scholarly article on the subject, does not. I testified that Leslie, although legally sane, was essentially suffering from a *folie en famille*. (*Folie a deux* is a term for shared psychotic delusion, wherein the partner of a dominant psychotic individual assumes the same delusional system in order to maintain the relationship.) Sometimes small groups, or "families", share their leader's delusional system, which is usually heavily apocalyptic in nature (for example, the Branch Davidians, People's Temple, or Heaven's Gate). Leslie did stab Mrs. La Bianca in the back. Was the blameworthiness of her action, however, lessened by the fact that she was high on LSD at the time or that Mrs. La Bianca may already have been dead by the time Leslie stabbed her?

The nature of the punishment is the question here. Was Leslie rehabilitated after the several years she had done in prison before her retrial? Yes. Did she represent an ongoing danger to society? No. Was she punished enough? This is the relevant question because every couple of years that Leslie has come up for parole, she has been routinely denied. I testified that, under the influence of this charismatic leader, Leslie had a diminished capacity to harbor malice and to form a premeditated intent to kill; therefore, the eight years that she had already served should have made her eligible for parole. If one views incarceration as punishment, she should never get out; however, if one wants her to lead a constructive life, then this intelligent and genuinely remorseful young woman should be given the opportunity to devote her life to the service of others. Should she be in prison or not? (My views about the others who were convicted are quite different.)

There were other lesser known trials that I shall not describe in great detail which also raised interesting issues. The following case was the subject of a book written by the subject's defense attorney. A longtime male secretary/companion of a socially prominent San Francisco "pillar of the community" killed his late employer's widow, his subsequent employer, while on a cruise ship. Prior to the trip to Alaska, he had gotten the lady (then under sedation in recovery from surgery) to change her will so that the majority of her fortune would be left to him rather than to the Catholic Church. (Actually, the Church paid for his excellent legal defense by giving him $300,000 in return for his waiver of rights to the estate, just in case he would be found innocent and the new will would be valid.) Having power of attorney, shortly before the ship left San Francisco, he had written a check for $100,000 to his lover of 20 years (a retired Greek Orthodox priest) and $50,000 to the priest's son. As one might expect, this case created quite a stir in San Francisco society. Norway, the country of the ship's registration, refused to prosecute; therefore, our federal government launched an extensive, costly investigation. I was retained by the Department of Justice because the defendant, a chronic alcoholic, claimed that if he had perpetrated the crime, which he claimed not to recall, it would have been during an alcoholic fugue state that would have rendered him not legally sane. Only after a year of preparation for the case did the department inquire of the Coast Guard as to the probable location of the ship at the time of the killing. It was in Canadian waters; the United States had no jurisdiction. Canada agreed to prosecute, and the defendant unsuccessfully fought extradition. The Canadian Crown Prosecutor retained me, since I had done so much work on the case already.

Although Canada and the United States share the tradition of British Common Law, their criminal judicial proceedings are quite different from one another. (Canada's proceedings are actually closer to Britain's.) In Canada, the judge plays a more active role, and the attorneys are required to "put all their cards on the table". To my amazement, as a witness for the prosecution, I was told to disclose openly and privately to the defense attorney what I was going to say in court. The trial was much shorter than it would have been in the United States. I considered the defendant sane, and he was convicted of first degree murder. As has become increasingly apparent to the public, American trials are often about how much information can be kept out of the courtroom and not about how much data can be brought in. As a scientist, I feel that more data facilitates the decision-making process, although one need question their reliability and validity.

I shall describe a personal encounter with a probably all-too-common violation of legal ethics that likely had lethal consequences. (No one will ever know.) A small-time, self-described "professional strong-arm robber" made up in volume what he lacked in profit margin. He robbed little one-proprietor stores in small towns, traveling all over the country to do so, never robbing more than one in any given area. His crimes were not large enough to warrant major time behind bars; besides, small town police departments have little capacity to investigate. Crimes were geographically distant and, thus, not associated by police. He had earned enough over the past 20 years to "work" nine months a year and travel in luxury the other three. This man was eventually apprehended for the killing of a gas station attendant. Upon questioning, he confessed offhandedly to me that the killing had been only the most recent of over 40 that he had committed in the last two years! He had discovered that it was "easier to kill people" after robbing them. For the first 18 years of his criminal career, he never shot anyone. Then, he encountered a brave but foolish elderly antique store proprietor who refused to hand over money even after he shot a bullet into the floor to show her what he would do if she didn't give him the money. She still refused, and he shot her. His continued killing of almost all robbery victims likely came from stored hostility, which was released once fantasy had become reality, as has also occurred in some Vietnam veterans who later engaged in violent crimes. Once hostile fantasies are *actualized*, it is difficult to "put the genie back in the bottle".

I informed the "small business killer's" lawyer that his client had no psychiatric defense and that he was a *serial killer*. Despite the information, the attorney pursued a *not guilty* plea by alibi, producing two witnesses who "vouched" for having seen the accused elsewhere at the time of the crime. I, of course, was bound by lawyer-client (not doctor-patient) privileged communication. The defendant was acquitted, presumably to continue the same pattern of behavior. Although defense attorneys are obligated to try to get the best possible outcomes for their clients, once a client has confessed to a crime, it seems legally unethical to try to get the person acquitted. I think that most criminal lawyers prefer that their clients not tell them details of a crime actually committed. I believe that this lawyer should have told his client, "I now know the whole true story. You'll have to find yourself another lawyer to whom you can lie if you wish." When does the withholding of information become unethical? The boundaries are not always clear.

Some cases for which I was asked to consult had outcomes that proved to be more gratifying than others. There was the man who hired a pricey, first class attorney (who, in turn, hired me as a potential expert witness) to defend his wife after she had tried to hire a "hit man" to kill him. This wealthy man had married a very attractive woman (Veda) of very low intelligence, whom I found to have an IQ of 70. (I had learned in the military that it takes an IQ of about 80 to get through basic training. In other words, she was borderline mentally retarded.) In addition to being attractive, Veda had good social skills and was, therefore, able to hide her disability rather successfully. Being of scant mental resources, she sought advice from a crystal ball-gazing fortune teller and from her sister as well. Unfortunately, her intelligent and nefarious sister had been colluding with the fortune teller to con Veda out of her potential inheritance. The fortune teller told Veda that her husband was gay and having an affair with a man. The husband, in truth, had a very effeminate manner. (Both macho and, conversely, effeminate manners have poor correlation with either heterosexuality or homosexuality.) This story was reinforced by her sister, who told her that since her husband was a two-timing faggot, he deserved to be killed. Veda agreed to hire the hit man, but the one she attempted to hire turned out to be a policeman in civilian clothes. He arrested her immediately. Veda was acquitted of the charge of soliciting killing for hire and went back to living with her loving, effeminate heterosexual husband. The sister and fortune teller were convicted of conspiracy to commit murder.

Another time, I was asked by the police to identify which of several suspects might have been responsible for the serial killing of several young women, since I had examined quite a few serial killers. The prime suspect was a young man, Hank, in his early 20s who, in my opinion, did not possess the characteristics of a serial murderer. I was quite convinced that he had a strong conscience and was neither a sexual deviant nor a psychopath. Hank had empathic, concerned relationships with other people, including women. Nothing in his dating history seemed out of the ordinary. Trying to gather more information about the young man's upbringing, I interviewed his father. (His mother was deceased.) Unlike Hank, his father was bizarre. He impressed me as a misogynist whose remarks about women were sexually charged. He continually boasted of vicarious enjoyment of his son's sexual activities with young women friends, at the same

GEORGE FREEMAN SOLOMON, M.D.

time expressing enormous hostility toward women as a result of his
ex-wife, who had left him long before her death. Since Hank and his
father had a good deal of interaction, I thought that the clues that
had lead to Hank might also have been relevant to his father. I told
the police that Hank was unlikely to be the perpetrator, but that his
father could be, and I prompted them to start digging around his
father's house. Fortunately, there was enough evidence to get a search
warrant for the home and its rural surroundings. A dozen or so skeletons
were dug up, and Hank's father was convicted as the serial killer.

Then there was helping to solve a castration murder. Photos of
the corpse revealed a muscular young man (genitalia neatly removed)
with a crew cut and a number of tattoos, including a Marine Corps
emblem. The day after the killing, a note was found attached to the
door of the young man's apartment from the victim's mother stating
that she would attempt to find the victim's killer and, if successful,
would castrate him, kill him, and cut him into little pieces. I was
asked to interview the mother, but I thought it would be better for
the interview to be conducted by a police officer so she would not be
wary of being "psyched out". Since police officers usually do "just the
facts Ma'am" types of interviews, I asked for an opportunity to coach
the police officer who would be doing the interview. The police officer turned out to be an extremely handsome man in his 30s whom
the mother attempted to seduce during the subsequent interview. Before the attempted seduction, he found out that the mother had been
promiscuous, but for most of the victim's childhood she had lived
with a wealthy lesbian woman who "kept" her, and then she resumed
her heterosexual promiscuity. She also reported having had a very
close relationship with her son, who would discuss his sex life, which
allegedly did not include anything bizarre or perverse. After hearing this
report, I told the police that, in light of the highly sexualized relationship that the mother had established with people in general and probably with her son, and in view of the ambivalence he must have felt
toward her, "I think that you should be searching for a *woman* perpetrator, particularly a woman into 'S & M' [sadomasochistic] sex."

There was a lucky break in the case. One of the investigating police officers was dating a young woman, who told him that she had once been at a party with the victim. She had been there alone, and the victim had offered her a ride home. She accepted and, as they were passing a trailer park, he asked, "Would you mind if we swing in for a moment because I'm having an affair with a married woman who lives there, and if her husband is away she'll have a light on in a certain window that means I can come back. If the light is on, I'll drop you off in town and come back and see her." As it turned out, the light was on, and the victim in a gentlemanly way drove this young lady home, presumably then to return to the trailer house.

The woman who lived in the trailer house was married with a three-year-old child and said that she knew nothing of the victim. I advised the police to do whatever investigation of her that they possibly could. The police found out that, some months previously, this woman, Sybil, had gone to the emergency room of the county hospital bleeding from many lacerations in her vagina. She claimed that she had been waylaid and gang raped, unable to identify her assailants. The physician in the emergency room, however, had been highly suspicious of her story, since she did not have bruises, and the lacerations were very neat, sharp cuts. The physician had speculated in her chart that she had been masturbating with a dagger. Upon learning this, I said to the police, "It sounds like you've found your murderer." Both Sybil and her husband, Toby, were taken into custody for questioning, but could not be charged without further evidence.

Sybil adamantly refused to talk about anything; however, Toby finally buckled because of some sense of guilt, finally confessing that he and his wife had committed the crime. Toby agreed to a psychiatric interview. An amusing incident occurred immediately after that initial interview. We had been taken to a cell in an apparently unpopulated area of the jail for the several-hour interview. When it was over, I called out, "Guard." No one came. I yelled, "Guard, Guard!" louder. No response. I tried banging on the bars to no avail. Realizing my desperation at this predicament, Toby began to laugh; soon I was laughing, too. Two hours later, I scolded the guard who had finally arrived, "What kind of jail is this when a doctor is left unguarded and locked up alone with a castration murderer?!" (Confidentiality was not an issue, since Toby had confessed.)

Toby and Sybil had been involved in 'S & M' and group sex, often involving just one other man. Toby would feel very guilty about enjoying sex with the man, which he could only have in three-way or group situations. I asked, "Don't you think there is a big difference between sucking a cock and cutting one off?" He replied, "No. They're both wrong." Tending to get bored with previous acts, Sybil and Toby would escalate their sex behaviors for thrills. Sometimes, they had "standard sex", but for sadomasochistic behaviors they took vast amounts of amphetamine drugs. Illegal amphetamine tablets seized at the house were analyzed to contain three mg each. Toby was on a regular dose of six to nine mg of amphetamine per day and had taken the enormous amount of 60 mg prior to the crime. Toby said that he would be unable to describe his sexual exploits unless he were sexually aroused by a high dose of amphetamine. He consented to being given amphetamines in a hospital setting, but anticipated that he might not be able to get into a sex mood in that environment; perhaps pornography would help. With county purchase order in hand, I went to a porno bookstore. My criterion for purchase was not anything that was even remotely arousing to me but only the most revolting, disgusting, and horrible sadomasochistic and pedophilic pornography I could find. When I presented the clerk with $60 worth of pornography, asking him to sign a payment voucher for reimbursement, he was certain that I was an agent trying to get him arrested. I reassured him that this was a legitimate county purchase order for which he would be paid.

Before proceeding with the amphetamine interview, I inquired of one of the leading psychopharmacologists in the country as to how much amphetamine I could safely give to a healthy young man, who no longer had an addictive tolerance to the drug. He said 30 mg would be quite safe. Just before administering the drug, I showed the pornography to Toby, who turned away with disgust. With crash cart (for medical emergencies), male nurse, and burly sheriff's deputy present, I boldly gave Toby 40 mg of amphetamine. He soon grabbed at the pornography, had an erection, tried to grab and grope the male nurse, the sheriff's deputy, and me. He was sexually excited in a completely undifferentiated way. He told of heat sterilizing hat pins by flame and inserting them through Sybil's breasts. It turned out that they had felt that they had done everything there was to do, until *Sybil* suggested the ultimate experience: a castration murder. Toby went along with it. Sybil had had prior contact with the victim (Toby had not), but hadn't seen him in a long enough time such that there would be no tie-in to them. They went over to his house and, while giving him a back rub, Sybil signaled Toby to bludgeon him over the head with a hammer. The victim's genitals were removed and played with at home, but Toby didn't find them much fun. He eventually led the police to the location of the genitals, which had been buried in a coffee can at the base of a tree. One reason that Toby confessed was because his wife was having sex with their three-year-old daughter, of which he disapproved but was unable to prevent.

Perhaps I should have omitted the last disgusting case; however, on a sexual as well as aggressive level, it illustrates the depth of man's and woman's potential for depravity. Of course, such depravity can exist beyond the privacy of home—in Nazi Germany, the former Soviet Union, Vietnam, Bosnia, the Spanish Inquisition (in the name of religion). The case also illustrates some too-little-appreciated dangers of stimulant drugs.

The hope of mankind lies not only in successfully controlling hostility but also in promoting identification with one's fellow man. I refer to *mankind*, beyond the sociobiology of tribalism, a continuing scourge of society. Again, *those who empathize do not victimize.* Our failures in prevention and treatment of cruelty stem from indifference, ignorance, negligence, social irresponsibility, and vindictiveness. I believe that the human potentiality for good (based ultimately on the biology of social affiliative behaviors) is as great as that for evil. I also like to believe that the human's capacity for growth and healing is greater than his or her proclivity for violence.

CHAPTER VIII

NO MONOPOLY ON EVIL: VIETNAM

Where was my heart to flee for refuge from my heart?
Whither was I to fly, where I would not follow? In what
place should I not be prey to myself?

St. Augustine
Confessions, Book IV

Sam was a husky, 18-year-old, active duty Marine, who had been transferred to a Naval general hospital following a serious suicide attempt after six months of service in Vietnam. Upon a second attempt at wrist slashing in the hospital, he was transferred to the Palo Alto Veterans Administration Hospital, which was superior in security and management of more seriously disturbed patients. I was there at that time doing research on the effects of stress on immunity in rodents and on immunologic abnormalities in psychiatric patients. An increasing number of young, relatively recently discharged Vietnam veterans were being admitted to the hospital.

A resident presented this difficult case to me for supervisory help. In contrast to his well-adjusted older brother, Sam's parents had characterized him as a restless and easily frustrated child, prone to temper tantrums and poor performance in school. He had been occasionally brutalized by his alcoholic father. Sam felt that he was, in turn, a bad influence on others; for example, at the age of eight he had felt personally responsible for the fall and subsequent death of a playmate.

Along with puberty came an increasing preoccupation with death, dying, and sadomasochistic fantasies. Sam described sticking pins into his arms, ingesting diluted weed and rat poison, and drinking the blood of a dead cat "to see how much I could take". At the age of 16, he dropped out of high school. Sam's girlfriend of three years had left him prior to his tour of military duty because she had become scared of him.

Sam was guarded, suspicious, and denying of any existence of despondency—answering "fine" to any questions asked about his feelings. He would say that nothing remarkable had occurred in regard to his experiences in Vietnam. In spite of the administration of anti-psychotic drugs at both hospitals, Sam remained provocative, impulsive, and suicidal. He demanded immediate release from the facility. Following another suicidal episode at our hospital (his life spared by a male nursing assistant, who heroically managed to wrest a razor blade from his hands as he was attempting to slash his throat), I became determined to find out what was troubling the young man. In so doing, I hoped to teach the treating resident about the use of a valuable tool for retrieving suppressed (conscious but not verbalized) information: so-called "truth serum". (Psychopaths *can* lie under truth serum, but it is a bit harder to do so. Deluded psychotics truthfully report their delusions. Mute patients talk.)

"Truth serum" refers to a relatively short-acting (two-to four-hour) and inhibition-reducing sedative (usually sodium amobartibal, Amytal®), which is administered in narcoanalytic interviews. Such interviews were found to be useful in World War II and the Korean War. A "crash cart" replete with intubation and other medical supplies is kept at hand for any complications stemming from intravenous barbiturates, such as oversedation and laryngeal spasm. (Fortunately, I have never had to use the cart.) Because barbiturates cause patients to get very drowsy, I have found a double whammy approach to narcoanalytic interviews to be more useful. The sedative is first administered to produce a drunken-like state of disinhibition, followed by an injection of methamphetamine hydrochloride ("speed")—a highly arousing substance that promotes the urge to speak. Such a combination can be rather pleasant and is sometimes used by drug addicts. [My ability to do narcoanalytic interviews later proved useful in some forensic cases, but was eventually hampered by the inaccessibility of certain stimulant drugs. Both the intravenous forms of methamphetamine and methylphenidate (Ritalin®), a similar-acting but milder drug that had to be used in larger doses, were removed from the market. I now do these interviews by giving about 40 milligrams of oral dextroamphetamine until it begins to take hold, and then giving the intravenous amobarbital.] Over the course of five to ten minutes, the sodium amobarbital is slowly administered intravenously. During this time, emotionally charged topics are avoided and patients are asked to count backwards from 100. The altered state of consciousness is recognized when the patient's speech becomes blurred and thickened, and when he or she can no longer recall his or her own identity. At this point, a bolus (quick entire dose) of methamphetamine (20 milligrams) is injected through the same intravenous needle.

With assurance that he could speak without self-incrimination, Sam consented to the narcoanalytic interview. Under the influence of the drugs, he unleashed an outpouring of feelings: fear of his father, hostile childhood fantasies, enlistment in the Marines "to get the hate out of my system", rebelliousness in basic training toward provocative drill instructors, minor infractions of military rules, and pride over his "40 confirmed Viet Cong kills". He seemed to like his time of service in Vietnam until the following incident occurred. Sam had befriended a 14-year-old Vietnamese girl, with whom he spent most of an entire day. "She was a nice kid, a virgin, no VC (Viet Cong). I would never have tried anything with her; she wasn't even developed. We just walked around." The next day, Sam's corporal, threatening him with court martial for repeated rule violations, ordered him to shoot the 14-year-old for having rebuffed the corporal's sexual advances. Reluctantly and fearfully, he complied with the order—shooting the girl in the abdomen, killing her. Sam became intensely disturbed by this event. Later that day, he provoked a fight with the corporal; whereupon, the corporal drew a bayonet and Sam shot him—making it look as if the corporal had been killed by the Viet Cong (fragging). Soon thereafter, Sam was hospitalized for depression of psychotic degree. "How can I ever live with myself knowing what I have done?" he pleaded under drug-induced disinhibition. I was utterly appalled by the story and asked that any veterans who seemed to have difficulty dealing with something about Vietnam be sent to me for special evaluation.

I told the resident, "Now that you know what's really bothering Sam, you are in a much better position to help him" (unfortunately, this turned out to be untrue). Sam began to settle down, socialize tentatively, and make plans for his release from the hospital. After going on two weekend passes to visit his family, he spent the next several weeks at the hospital making some progress. Nonetheless, he still obsessed about death and made yet another dramatic attempt at throat cutting, in which he was chased across the grounds by two psychiatric residents and a nurse, following the denial of a request for a longer pass. After a one-day visit with his father, from which he returned in good spirits, a week-long pass was granted him along with precautionary notes to Sam and his parents. During this time his parents attempted to support and reassure him while he spoke of wanting to die for his transgressions in Vietnam. He called the hospital and was urged to return by the nursing staff and fellow patients. Later, after talking with his girlfriend about their pending engagement, he was left alone at her home with access to her father's unloaded guns and shot himself in the head with a 0.22 caliber shell that he had been carrying on his person. He never regained consciousness.

The second deeply disturbed patient that I evaluated narcoanalytically was a tall, slim, 26-year-old computer operator named Bill, who had been admitted to our hospital several days after a suicide gesture that included a superficial laceration of one wrist and the ingestion of a few proprietary sleeping tablets. Having been unemployed for the first nine months after completing six years of service in the Army, he took to working almost daily for up to 10 hours a day. His suicide gesture followed an argument with his girlfriend, resulting in her moving out of the home they shared.

Bill's family had moved about a great deal during his childhood because his father had been a military officer. His mother was a successful engineer. Bill's parents separated when he was in the 11th grade, during a rocky point in his father's career. At the time of hospitalization, he had had little contact with his father or 16-year-old brother. Beginning in early childhood, Bill would routinely dress in his mother's clothing, which he combined with masturbation after he reached puberty. He was ashamed of this behavior, which he kept well-guarded, and maintained an active heterosexual life. At the age of 18, Bill enlisted in the Army, volunteering for airborne and Special Forces training. He served three tours in Vietnam with elite Green Beret units, reaching the grade of sergeant E6; however, during the third tour, his performance deteriorated markedly. He began provoking conflicts with superior officers until he was relegated to a minor administrative position in a rear unit and was ultimately discharged for having a "character disorder".

Bill showed such evasiveness following hospitalization that he was released after three days only to return four days later because of an inability to function. Eventually, he requested a narcoanalytic interview to assist in getting things off his chest about which he was afraid to talk. During the interview, Bill reported pride in his first two tours of duty in Vietnam, feeling manly and heroic in his daring exploits and efforts to stop the Communists in Asia. On his third tour, however, he became horrified by the futility and cruelty of the war to which he desensitized himself with the use of amphetamines (up to 100 mg a day). Being a medic for "counterinsurgency" forces, drugs were readily accessible to him.

One night, while on a secret river patrol in the Mekong Delta, "high" on amphetamines and having been sleepless for 26 hours, Bill became jumpy. Upon hearing a noise, he turned and suddenly opened automatic weapon fire on an accompanying boat—killing over a dozen South Vietnamese soldiers from his own unit and wounding two American advisors. Their deaths and injuries were assumed due to enemy attack. Bill's role in the incident was never questioned. Obsessed with guilt and having received no punishment, Bill began sabotaging his own military career. Following discharge, Bill felt that he could only justify living by serving others. He befriended a disturbed girl, who was emotionally demanding while sexually rejecting, in order to save her. He considered himself a failure, this view reinforced by a brief and failed attempt at college, and his transvestism recurred.

Following the drug interview, Bill became more respectful of ward rules, formed an excellent working alliance with his therapist, and participated in group meetings. While continuing with outpatient psychotherapy, he obtained a challenging job and attempted to assume responsibility for his younger brother.

The third patient whose trauma was revealed through the amobarbital-methamphetamine procedure was Lee, a 24-year-old African-American construction worker. Lee had been admitted to the Surgery Service of the VA Hospital for persistent and increasingly incapacitating pain and hyperesthesia (excessive or pathologic sensitivity of the skin) in the scar of an abdominal wound he had sustained in Vietnam nearly two years earlier. Surgical opinion maintained, as it had judged the year prior, that there was no organic basis for this pain and recommended transfer to the Psychiatry Service was recommended. Following transfer, Lee was treated with a variety of antianxiety and antipsychotic drugs to no avail. His behavior was compliant, apathetic, and somewhat withdrawn, and he continued to deny any possibility that emotional factors may have played a role in his symptomatology.

During the narcoanalytic interview, Lee disclosed a traumatic discovery that he had made just prior to entering the service: the man whom he had considered his father all his life had actually been his stepfather, and he had been born out of wedlock. Lee had always felt that his father favored his younger siblings, who, unlike him, did not have to earn money to buy their own clothes and were given an opportunity to learn trades. In spite of this distressing new knowledge, Lee had no apparent difficulties in the Army—although he disliked service in Vietnam, combat in particular. He was a private person but had one confidante, his lieutenant, and one close friend with whom he spent much off-duty time, the platoon medic.

One day, Lee told another soldier to throw a grenade into a bunker, but it bounced back, killing the soldier and two others. Lee reported feeling much guilt over this incident. A few days later he was shot in the abdomen. His medic friend cared for him and helped load him onto the "med evac" helicopter, at the usual considerable risk to his own life. While doing so, the medic was shot and severely wounded in the lower extremities. Lee was very reluctant to be evacuated from Vietnam and never learned whether the legs of his friend, with whom he had lost contact, had been saved. He expressed a great deal of guilt and sense of responsibility for what happened in Vietnam, remarking, "I deserve to suffer." Somewhat surprisingly, the hyperesthesia persisted during the drug interview.

The interview indicated that Lee had been suffering from depression, with guilt aggravating his already low sense of self-esteem. He was placed on antidepressant medication and given psychotherapy aimed at helping him ventilate resentment toward his stepfather and develop a more sympathetic point of view *vis-à-vis* the events in Vietnam. Lee became markedly more animated and participated actively in the ward community. Physical discomfort subsided, and with support from hospital services, he found employment much more to his liking than heavy manual labor.

Psychiatric casualties as a result of Vietnam were initially reported to be few, the low rate being attributed to lessons learned from other wars—early treatment of mental distress, prompt medical care near the front after helicopter evacuation, shorter combat experiences, frequent periods of rest and relaxation, and, especially, the fixed one-year tour of duty. This minimization of psychiatric problems proved to be utterly misleading. Of 50 random psychiatric admissions of Vietnam veterans to the Palo Alto VA Hospital in 1970-71, only eight had been identified with emotional problems while in service. Of these 50 patients, 60% were seriously ill, receiving diagnoses of psychotic illness (the most common being paranoid schizophrenia). Many had been referred to the VA Hospital through police rather than medical channels.

Several factors prevented early recognition of psychiatric distress in Vietnam. Some men complaining of emotional symptoms were simply sent back into the field by commanding or medical officers. More typically, "acting out" behavior (indicative of emotional conflict) led to disciplinary measures, particularly dishonorable discharges for character disorders. Frequent periods of safety slowed down the pace of accumulated stress and allowed soldiers to maintain emotional detachment as a means of coping.

Wartime-related psychological syndromes, such as "survivor guilt", have been reported as long ago as the Civil War. Yet, the sorts of stresses unique to Vietnam could cause psychological traumas of an intensity greater than those witnessed in other wars. For example, American soldiers were not sent over in military units, but were rotated individually for a year's tour of duty, resulting in very little *esprit de corps*. Newly arrived soldiers were distrusted as "green" and undependable. Young, lower echelon, command officers were often not well-trained for the peculiar guerrilla war being fought in the villages and exhibited poor judgment, causing the troops to lose faith in their leadership. Furthermore, the identity of the enemy was unclear, with a blurring of distinctions among North Vietnamese soldiers, actual civilians, and the civilian-based Viet Cong (which included women and young people). There was even ambivalence about Indochinese allies.

Unlike most wars, the goal of the Vietnam war was not about the recovery of territory. In fact, hills would be taken and given back repeatedly, solely for the purpose of killing. It was a war in which body counts seemed to be the criterion of success. Atrocities became commonplace. People did things either at the behest of or in defiance of their superiors that they would never have done elsewhere. Going against one's conscience to commit an act of major consequence would understandably result in a guilt-induced psychiatric reaction. The absence of a sense of righteousness and meaning grounded in strong basic moral principles for which our nation was fighting, coupled with the younger generation's inherent tendency toward skepticism of the establishment, could exacerbate feelings of guilt (for example, "I'm ashamed for what I did, like throwing grenades into hooches not knowing who was in there"). Such guilt I consider "realistic", in contradistinction to the more "neurotic" guilt of survivorship, whereby happiness at remaining alive is tantamount to being glad that friends

were killed. Since guilt for doing atrocious things (like wanton killing of civilians) is "appropriate", it is harder to treat; psychiatrists are
trained to treat illness. I actually felt that many guilt-ridden veterans
were "healthier" than those who bragged of "wasting Gooks". ("Gook"
is a pejorative term for a Vietnamese, particularly a North Vietnamese, person.) When the President committed the United States to
progressive withdrawal, soldiers became even more reluctant to risk
their lives and kill the "enemy".

Meanwhile, the war had become increasingly unpopular back
home, leaving soldiers to feel more like martyrs, victims, pariahs, or
criminals than heroes, leading to resentment and bitterness. Peers,
especially those involved with antiwar groups, could not empathize
with experiences in Vietnam. Jobs were hard to find after coming
home. Vietnam vets were often considered to be high risk for insta-
bility, and many of them had been called to serve before having the
opportunity to acquire necessary trade skills, educational credentials,
or job experience. For instance, a VA representative in St. Louis pointed
out that African-American veterans had a higher unemployment rate
and lower average wages than African-Americans of similar age and
educational background who did not serve. Especially important is
the fact that many veterans returned with markedly altered views toward our country and society. The horror, corruption, devastation,
and futility experienced in Vietnam, combined with disillusionment
with what had been taught by parents, schools, and military authorities, led to a profound sense of alienation in some vets. Faith in the
integrity and credibility of the establishment may have been shat-
tered. Moreover, many of those who served in Vietnam were socio-
economically, and possibly emotionally, disadvantaged at the outset.
The educated elite and wealthy could obtain prolonged school ex-
emptions, prepare convincing erudite statements of conscientious ob-
jection, or obtain paid-for medical or psychiatric opinions suggesting
reasons for disqualification from the draft. Perhaps the stronger copers
were the conscientious objectors who went to prison or fled to Canada.
Clever soldiers might have manipulated their way into being stationed in the U.S., Europe, Korea, or safer posts in Vietnam.

In light of all these unfortunate circumstances, it did not surprise me that in addition to seeing soldiers with "war neuroses" (or what would later be called acute posttraumatic stress disorder), more than half of the vets that I was seeing were addicted to opiates (namely, heroin). Heroin was readily available in Vietnam toward the end of the war, after 1967 but especially after 1969, and I suspect possibly as a deliberate act by the North Vietnamese. Physical addiction to the drug was made even greater by the fact that the heroin was cheap and strong—97% pure, unlike good street heroin in the United States, which is 40% pure at best. (Marijuana was also of a stronger variety in Vietnam than the domestic.) A $10 per day habit in Vietnam would be roughly equivalent to a $200 per day habit at home. Official figures in 1971 stated that 10% of the troops in Vietnam were addicted to heroin; the actual rate may have been double. A typical patient of ours reported that about 35 out of 96 men in his unit were shooting up.

Besides the sheer presence of a drug (barring prior experience with hard drugs), stress and personality factors are involved in creating drug addiction. I don't really believe in an "addictive type" personality *per se*, although people who tend to use denial as a defense (that is, pretending that what they see isn't really there) and those who have some difficulty in coping seem to be more likely candidates for addiction. The availability of the heroin and the stress that the GIs were under was so great that their addiction may not have required many predisposing personality factors.

I asked a young addict how he began to use heroin in Vietnam. The man openly described being part of a team that interrogated Viet Cong prisoners. They would take the prisoners up in helicopters and inform them that, if they didn't divulge information regarding Viet Cong activities, they'd be thrown out. The prisoners would, as expected, provide the information—and be thrown out of the helicopters anyway. "I simply found it easier to throw people out of helicopters when I was loaded on heroin," he confessed. Another young addict was involved in ferrying ARVN (Army of the Republic of Vietnam, allied) troops by helicopter to dangerous areas of operation in the Delta. Frequently, these soldiers were reluctant to land and had to be forced from the "choppers" sometimes by beating their hands as they clung to the runners. Two of the vet's friends were killed by bullets from U.S. M16 rifles, having been shot by resentful ARVN troops after they had been landed unwillingly. The vet turned to heroin in order to be able to keep flying, while many of his friends refused flying status. Once gung-ho and resentful of antiwar demonstrations at home, the young vet became militantly antiwar.

This type of story brings up a crucial and often overlooked point. In some ways, the use of drugs by our troops was advantageous to the military. Drugs like marijuana and heroin have a tranquilizing effect, enabling some men to face otherwise unbearable situations and handle powerful emotions of fear, guilt, rage, and even meaningless boredom. Often I heard, "If I wasn't stoned, I'd have split." As such, sometimes these drugs enabled, rather than interfered with, functioning. While under the influence, troops may have been less likely to rebel when commanded by their officers to do otherwise unacceptable things. Often soldiers thought that they were taking cocaine, but in reality they were becoming addicted to heroin. The pusher was often a "papa san", or family man, with whom the lonely soldier formed an affectionate parent-surrogate relationship. A drug-supplying papa san of one of our VA patients had offered his daughter's hand in marriage, considered a great honor. On the contrary, another of our patients reported killing his "boy san", who "burned" him by not returning with the heroin for which he had been given money.

Once removed from the stresses of Vietnam and the availability of heroin, many soldiers—even those quite physically addicted—were able to get off the drug on their own or at the hospital. Some of these vets were helped by the fact that they had never been part of a drug subculture and, therefore, did not even know how to "cop" drugs off the street. Conversely, the heaviness of the habit combined with the ignorance of the game of hustling may have made the adjustment more difficult for some vets, who even reenlisted to return to Vietnam for inexpensive, powerful heroin. Still other vets, troubled by distressing memories, became heroin addicts *after* returning to the States.

Ironically, the VA was not legally permitted to treat heroin addicts! Alcoholism, however, had been a major condition treated at VA hospitals for some years. (Congress had always been supportive of alcohol treatment through the VA, not only because there was a moral judgment against the use of illegal substances but also because Congress has many recovering as well as active alcoholic members.) *Our* response to the pressing need for drug treatment at the Palo Alto VA Hospital was to create a unit specifically designed for heroin-addicted Vietnam vets (the first of its kind) and to conduct "stealth treatment". We never put down a diagnosis of heroin addiction in the patients' records, only "anxiety reaction" or some other psychiatric term. We would never even mention heroin until later events occurred necessitating such disclosure. In our drug abuse treatment unit, we found that nothing short of a comprehensive program, including availability of methadone maintenance, psychotherapeutic care, and rehabilitation services, would be effective in treating heroin addiction. The three phases of our program, lasting 12-16 weeks, included "cleaning up", "getting your head on straight", and "learning to live in the real world". After discharge, those on methadone maintenance would return every morning for medication, once a week for social therapeutic (that is, peer group) involvement, and monthly for progress evaluation and planning. Our staff worked one-on-one with the patients. Without such programs, the vast majority of patients would relapse even if withdrawn from the drug to which they are addicted. [Nowadays, so much later, many VA centers (including the Sepulveda VA Medical Center where I worked in Los Angeles) have good programs that face curtailment.]

Drug treatment programs needed to be legitimized and funded, and these stories had to be told. Since the psychiatric residents were not responding to my nudging, I had to write up the cases myself. My first paper, coauthored with residents and ward chiefs, was entitled, "Three Psychiatric Casualties From Vietnam", which I promptly submitted to the *Archives of General Psychiatry*. (The *Archives* series, including the *Archives of Internal Medicine, Archives of Surgery,* and so forth, is published by the American Medical Association.) To my surprise, I received an immediate written response from the Editor, the late Daniel X. (Danny) Freedman (who later became one of my bosses at UCLA, as Executive Vice Chair of the Department of

Psychiatry under Jolly West). Considering the importance and time-liness of the piece that I had submitted, Dr. Freedman boldly took the Editor's prerogative of accepting it without delay, rather than sending it out for peer review. Both flattered and pleased, I waited for the article to be published. After several issues of the monthly journal had come out without it, I telephoned Dr. Freedman to voice my strong concern that, with the rise in psychiatric casualties from Vietnam, further delays in publication would be irresponsible. Dr. Freedman then explained that the report had been blocked from publication by the American Medical Association (AMA) on the grounds that it was not scientific but "political".

I was furious about the AMA's action and annoyed that I had not been previously informed. As is characteristic when pushed to my limits (fortunately, it takes quite a bit to get me there), I blew up. I told Dr. Freedman that if the paper did not appear in the next issue I would sue him, the *Archives*, and the AMA under the First Amendment to the Constitution because I had it in writing that the piece had been accepted, and I felt that I was being politically censored. The article *did* appear in the next issue. (Interestingly, Dr. Freedman and I, in spite of a good deal of contact later, never talked about what had happened.) What ensued was a great political ruckus over the paper. I had assumed that the press only followed reports published in the *New England Journal of Medicine* and, to some degree, in the *Journal of the American Medical Association* but *not* the *Archives*. The AMA had clearly understood better than I that the press would promptly pick up on my paper. Producers from the Chet Huntley-David Brinkley NBC evening news asked if I would discuss the issues in an interview format with Mr. Brinkley from the KRON television studio in San Francisco. Two short segments, aired on consecutive evenings, followed.

Next, producer Edwin Newman invited me to appear on his Sunday afternoon half-hour interview program. Out of great respect for Mr. Newman, I agreed and was interviewed in the San Francisco television studio while Mr. Newman was in New York. Then Australian National Television sent a crew to Palo Alto to do a story on my observations, since Australia, too, had sent troops to Vietnam.

Incidentally, I did not have to get permission from the VA to participate in these television segments because I was not a full-time employee of the VA (Stanford would only allow its faculty to have 5/8 of
their salary paid for by the VA in a symbiotic relationship that gave
Stanford some salary help while the VA benefitted from good clinical
care and resident supervision.) Thus, wearing the Stanford hat gave
me license to speak out publicly on topics for which the VA would
never have given me clearance.

Eventually, I was approached by the producer of the Dick Cavett
show, who wanted my participation in an interview and discussion
with some Vietnam vets on one of their 90-minute late night programs, nationally broadcast on ABC. I declined. The next call I received was from Dick Cavett himself inquiring as to why I had declined. I had told the producer that they should get an official representative from the VA to be the discussant, and the producer had
informed me that the VA had already been approached and had declined. Nonetheless, as strongly as I felt about the need to rally public
concern on behalf of the vets, I did not feel that the format of the
show (typically involving celebrity guests and Mr. Cavett's comic
monologues) was appropriate for this subject matter. I so told Mr.
Cavett. He assured me that it would be a very serious program and
that there would be no initial comic monologue. He also informed
me that in addition to the vets that they had secured, I would be free
to bring, at their expense, any Vietnam vet that I wished to join me on
the program. It was a deal.

Owing to my concern with heroin abuse in Vietnam (an article I
had written on the subject having just been published), I brought
with me to New York a Mexican-American vet—a nice, articulate
young man who was still receiving slow methadone detoxification. I
took along a bottle of methadone tablets and doled out his dose each
day of the trip. In light of his impending vacation, Mr. Cavett had to
tape two shows during one afternoon—ours, that was to be aired the
same evening, and another program the following evening.

Besides the Chicano whom I had brought, there were three other
Vietnam vets who would be appearing on the program. One was a

wheelchair-bound, ex-Marine lieutenant, who had become paraplegic after being shot in the spine. The highly decorated lieutenant represented "Vietnam Veterans Against the War", an organization that he had helped to found and lead since his return. Another was a Navy lieutenant, who had flown missions over (but not set foot on) Vietnam while serving on a carrier off the coast. He represented "Vietnam Veterans for a Just Peace" (a pro-war group). The third vet was a highly volatile, nonpolitical war supporter who responded to all questions with intractable hostility. He had been beating up Chinese people in Boston as surrogate "Gook bastards", since he could not find any Vietnamese.

I had anticipated having at least a brief meeting with Mr. Cavett prior to the taping to familiarize us with the issues that he wanted to discuss. Quite to the contrary, all he did was joke around and tell stories—keeping us *completely* off the topic of Vietnam—while we waited in the "Green Room" to go into the studio. Mr. Cavett brought me out alone first and interviewed me for about 20 minutes. I described the cases that I had encountered, pulling my punches with great care so as not to make any comments that could be construed as political or take any position about the war itself. I only slipped once in quoting something negative about former President Lyndon Johnson (Nixon was President at that time) and immediately apologized for mentioning politics, as it was not my area of expertise.

The vets were brought out and what ensued was an inevitable crossfire. At one point, the educated Marine and the Navy lieutenant got into a heavy entanglement over whether or not the war was worth fighting. None of the three vets that Mr. Cavett had invited was able to see each other's point of view, except that the violent one who sought out "Gooks" seemed to begin to question his own behavior as a result of the discussion. The exchange was so lively that Mr. Cavett deliberately ignored the "commercial break" sign as well as the producer's shaking fist. Finally, when the last commercial break rolled around, Mr. Cavett turned to me and asked, "We've certainly not exhausted the topic, have we?"

"We've barely scratched the surface."

"I think I'm not going to tape tomorrow night's scheduled program, and we'll go on again."

"What about your guests who are waiting to perform?"

"Screw that show business shit. I'll apologize and ask them to take a raincheck."

On camera, Mr. Cavett announced, "I want to apologize to my guests for tomorrow night and ask them to return another time because I feel the topic of Vietnam and what it is doing to people is much too critical at this time for us not to continue; therefore, I am going to take the liberty of asking tonight's guests to return again tomorrow night [actually meaning to stay on and do a taping for tomorrow night's show]." By now, the already irate producer was behind the camera jumping up and down, grimacing, and literally pulling out his hair. (Incidentally, "tomorrow night's guest", the renowned D'Amboise was justifiably pissed off.)

We took a 20-minute break before going on for another even more powerful hour and a half. (I always wondered if the audience noticed that we were wearing the same clothes two nights in a row.) During the break I remarked to Cavett, "I was just beginning to relax at the time of the last commercial when the show was almost over. You know, I'm not a performer and being in front of millions of people is making me very nervous." Mr. Cavett asserted, "Bullshit. You're calmer than practically any of my guests ever are. Performers are comfortable when they're scripted. When they have to be themselves, they're often throwing up behind stage because they're used to playing roles and sometimes don't even have a self to be." Mr. Cavett's absolutely superb interviewing skills had brought out so much highly charged material from the vets that I offered to arrange to have him lecture to psychiatric residents on interviewing techniques if he ever wanted to come to Stanford.

The Vietnam vet whom I had brought out had never been to New York; so, after the taping I took him out for dinner and theater, culminating in an 11 PM "Dick Cavett party" thrown by an old friend of mine. After watching the show and discussing its implications, we didn't get back to the hotel until nearly 3 AM. We were immediately ushered to the front desk by the doorman of the Park Lane Hotel. The clerk at the desk seemed excited, blurting out, "Where in the world have you been? The White House has called several times."

I answered, innocently, "Well, we went out."

He handed me a slip of paper and instructed, "Promptly at nine o'clock you are to call this White House number."

I called, as I was told to do so, at nine o'clock. A voice informed me, "The President [Nixon] has seen last night's program and wishes you to know of his [exact quote] *grave personal displeasure at your antiwar views.* [I had not even discussed the war *per se* or been directly antiwar!] The President also wishes you to know that, if you do not cancel your appearance on tonight's program, you will be required to sever all your connections with the U.S. government." The voice threatened explicitly, "This means you will be fired from the VA, and any VA or National Institute of Health grants you have will be canceled."

I made no effort to control my rage, "I am terribly sorry. The program has already been taped for broadcast. And the reason I am terribly sorry is that I have been robbed of the opportunity to tell the American people about this gross attempt at fascistic intimidation." Then I hung up, shaking. I had been pretty naive, not believing that this sort of thing could happen in the United States. I was also scared. Although my job was pretty secure as a Stanford faculty member (not yet tenured), the fact that my research was being jeopardized made me very nervous. Both Alfred Amkraut, my immunologist associate, and a lab assistant were being supported by federal grant money.

Anxious about my research funding and VA position, I went to see the Chairman of my department, David Hamburg. David had always demonstrated superb judgment in delicate matters and was gifted at negotiation. (For example, some years later, he negotiated the release of some Stanford anthropology students who were being held for ransom in Africa.) After explaining the whole situation to David, he said that he would think about it and asked me to come back in two days. When I came back, he reported, "I've discussed this matter with President Lyman [of Stanford University], who has pledged the full resources of the university to back you. If anything happens, Stanford will hire a top-notch law firm to represent you, and there will be no limit on the expense undertaken on your behalf because freedom of speech and academic freedom are being challenged."

"I don't want to be a *cause celebre.* I don't want to be a Dreyfus case. I just want to go on with my research."

"What did you expect me to do? I did the most I could."

I was beginning to relax because nothing seemed to be happening, and I was assuming that whoever had spoken to me from the White House had been bluffing. A couple of months later, I was called in to see the Director of the Palo Alto VA Hospital, a layperson for whom I had a great deal of respect. He spoke frankly, "George, if you promise on your word of honor not to reveal to the press anything that I say, I'll tell you what has transpired." I made that promise, which I feel is now immaterial, and was informed thus. Word had come from the White House to the Veterans Administration to fire me. The Chief Medical Officer of the VA, Wendell Musser, M.D., inquired as to why and was told that it was a result of my remarks on the Dick Cavett show. He asked what I had said and was told that a tape of the program could be made available for him to review. He did so. (Dr. Musser, whom I never have had the privilege of meeting, was a pathologist, a Republican political appointee, and a man of great principle.) After viewing the tape, in an act of integrity and personal courage, he evidently said, "Solomon was telling the truth. He was merely pointing out how troubled some of our returning vets are and trying to obtain appropriate help for them. I will resign in public protest before I fire him." I was hopeful that Dr. Musser's position would put the problem to rest.

Sometime thereafter, several months after the Cavett program, I was awakened from sleep at about 2 AM by a telephone call. "I am an investigator for a branch of the U.S. Government," the voice said quietly, "and I am calling you at some personal risk because it's possible that your phone is tapped. However, I happen to concur with what you have been saying and feel that you have the best interests of our vets at heart. I just wanted you to know that every aspect of your professional and *personal* life is being looked at by an agency of the United States government, possibly to be used against you for political purposes." The phone went "click". It was at that point that I developed acute galloping paranoia.

Subsequently, I was called to testify before a public joint meeting of the Senate Veterans Affairs Committee, under Senator Alan Cranston, and the House Committee on Alcohol and Drug Abuse, headed by Representative William Hughes (to the best of my recall). I was particularly impressed with the sensitivity and compassion of Representative Hughes, an admitted recovering alcoholic who had been sober for many years. Excerpts of my testimony were televised. Having had my fill of Executive Branch threats, I took full advantage of this opportunity and gave Congress an unedited version of the problems as I saw them. I told them about the helicopter incident. I even raised the question of whether or not the use of heroin was condoned to make such atrocities possible. I spared no details. Fortunately, it was not long after those hearings before the rescinding of the regulation that the VA could not treat drug addiction. Soon, there was a special appropriation of $8,000,000 to establish treatment units for addicted Vietnam vets. At last, our bootlegged VA program could be made official and obtain additional staffing.

Still personally anxious about the White House threat, I decided to enlist the help of good friend Theodore Baer, who had been a major figure in Senator Cranston's first campaign for Senate and in the Democratic party. I asked Ted to do me the favor of having the Senator call me personally. I told Senator Cranston the whole story. He said he would do what he could, but that his ability to accomplish anything might be limited because he was a Democrat, and the administration, Republican.

Several months of nervousness went by. I heard nothing. At last, I got a call from Senator Cranston, who told me that he had had several meetings with White House staff and had made a *quid pro quo* deal on my behalf. The whole thing had been done by John Erlichman. I had indeed been placed on Nixon's notorious "enemies list"; however, Erlichman promised to call off the dogs. Nothing further would happen. I could relax. (Subsequent psychoanalyst associate Helen Stein used to say that the most difficult base human emotion to overcome is retribution. Although I don't think of myself as a particularly vindictive person, I must admit that I am not completely free of retributive qualities; I was quite gleeful when Erlichman went to prison.)

I hooked up with a friend of mine from the University of California San Francisco, Dr. Mardi Horowitz, probably the leading American researcher on psychotherapy and still on the faculty of UCSF. Mardi had been seeing Vietnam vets at the San Francisco VA Medical Center, so we joined forces to write, "A Prediction of Delayed Stress Response Syndromes in Vietnam Vets". It seemed obvious to us (and later proved to be the case) that some psychiatric problems would not manifest themselves in Vietnam or immediately upon return but much later after a period of apparent relief. We were, indeed, prescient in our observations. (For years there were no books about psychiatric problems in Vietnam vets or about posttraumatic stress disorder, and now there are dozens. It amazes me that people did not see what was right before their eyes. It does not amaze me that later there was a bandwagon effect. My own library has 22 books on Vietnam vets and their problems.)

The lingering trauma with which many vets live is well-illustrated by an incident that occurred a few years ago (while I was doing psychoneuroimmunology research at UCLA and simultaneously serving as Chief of the Drug Dependency Treatment Center at the Sepulveda VA Medical Center). We took a group of 15 addicted vets by bus to a noon matinee showing of the film *Platoon* at a public theater. We had prepared the vets fully in advance of the excursion and made special arrangements for evening and night staff to be present, so that each patient could be accompanied one-on-one by a staff member. Fortunately, the theater was nearly empty. There is a scene in *Platoon* in which a woman, whose village is being burned, is standing with her young daughter; a soldier is about to kill them, but another stops him from doing so. One of the vets sitting behind me started screaming at the top of his lungs, "Kill the bitch! Kill the fucking

Gook bitch! Kill the kid! Kill 'em!" I went to him and said, "I think we'd better go out to the lobby for a few minutes."

After the film, we had a four-hour debriefing discussion of the film and our reactions to it. One of the vets told the group some things about which he felt guilty and was extremely distraught. A young non-Vietnam vet in his 20s from a middle class San Fernando Valley family, who was being treated for addiction to marijuana, tried to comfort him by saying, "I don't know what you're feeling bad about. It was just Gooks. Look how much trouble Gooks have caused. World War II, Gooks; Korean War, Gooks; Vietnam War, Gooks. So just don't feel so bad."

The fact that some Vietnam vets, even up to the present moment, have not dealt with the issues they encountered in Vietnam is demonstrated by the fact that in 1994, while I was supervising a Chief Resident, a vet named Mack told the resident that some things had happened to him in Vietnam that were deeply disturbing but so hideous that he could not bring himself to talk about them. I joined the resident in consultation with Mack, who accepted the opportunity to have a narcoanalytic interview in hopes that he might be able to talk under such circumstances. Mack was very guarded at first, even under the influence of the drug, telling us relatively innocuous things as a way of testing our reactions. Initially, he merely told us of having stolen a jeep for his own personal use, an occurrence that was quite commonplace. Mack gradually let down his guard and revealed what had been troubling him. Next came a survivor guilt-type story. Mack had tried to throw a grenade that bounced back off a tree—killing his only close friend, who died in his arms. Mack felt responsible for his friend's death and never made another friend.

There was only one other person whom Mack really cared for while in Vietnam—his girlfriend, the "mama san" of the local house of prostitution. This relationship added to his sense of prestige. Meanwhile, he had volunteered for assignment to an intelligence unit to ferret out Viet Cong spies. There was clear evidence that the women at his girlfriend's brothel had been pumping the American soldiers for information and feeding it to the Viet Cong. In an act of retribution,

Mack let his comrades kill all the women, but he felt that *he* should be the one to do away with the mama san because she had been his girlfriend. He felt compelled to prove that he would even be willing to kill his own girlfriend in order to retaliate against spies. The killing was brutal. The interview got progressively more grisly.

After recanting these horrors, Mack's psychological condition improved. (The resident's and mine deteriorated.) This case illustrates the aforementioned distinction between neurotic vs. realistic guilt. Mack had certainly not intended to kill his friend with a grenade. It was an accident. Nonetheless, the intense and unrealistic guilt that followed led to later destructive behavior that substantiated his own sense of guilt realistically. The two kinds of guilt, thus, became inextricably intertwined and exponential. Unresolved guilt, or the inability to reconcile past experiences with one's current life, may have a variety of self-destructive consequences, including posttraumatic stress disorder.

Primary symptoms of posttraumatic stress disorder include recurring intrusive thoughts and dreams, waves of painful emotional reexperience, and compulsive repetition of trauma-related behavior, with concomitant secondary signs such as impaired social relationships, aggressive and/or self-destructive behavior, and fear of uncontrollable hostile impulses. Posttraumatic stress disorder may follow a period of psychological detachment manifested in thought denial, emotional numbness, and constrained behavior. This detachment protects the psyche by suppressing intrusive images, feelings, and behavior; therefore, these warning signs may easily be mistaken for apparent adjustment. The disorder can be precipitated by the arousal of new conflicts, such as questioning the patriotic value of the war or feeling disappointment in homecoming. Paradoxically, a safe environment may promote the relaxation of defenses and, consequently, permit the emergence of intrusive traumatic memories.

A typical case of posttraumatic stress disorder can be described as follows. Zeb has been back from Vietnam for about three years. He has done ostensibly well, being able to get a job and to marry; however, Zeb feels somewhat estranged from his peers at work and does not discuss combat experiences with them. He has begun to have difficulty sleeping and is haunted by unwanted daytime images and combat nightmares (although not always the same one). These scenes commonly involve atrocities, whether or not he is involved in committing them. During the day, Zeb is often suspicious and, when frustrated or afraid, feels in great danger of losing control over his hostile and aggressive impulses. He has begun to conceal firearms for self-protection. Zeb is also afraid of going crazy and feels guilty about deriving pleasure from recurring imaginary acts of great physical violence. He suffers from startle reactions, psychosomatic symptoms (headaches, cramps), anxiety attacks, apathy, and depression.

Zeb "chips" (intermittently uses) heroin, as well as sedatives, to relieve his depression, anxiety, fear, and hostility. Difficulties with others have erupted as a result of his continual suspiciousness, moodiness, surly behavior, and demands to be taken care of. He makes frequent threats and alienates interested others. In an effort to ward off any reminders that might trigger intrusive thoughts or emotional turmoil, Zeb reacts defensively when asked about his past experiences. He becomes progressively more isolated. Vietnam veterans do not have the same security as "obsessional neurotics", who may dwell on the prospect of doing harm to others but have never actually done so. Vets know that such violence is possible and that it may be pleasurable as well as guilt-provoking. Past reality blurs the distinction between current fantasy and future possibility. Due to the shortened distance between impulse and act, self-restraint is harder to impose. The use of drugs further blurs distinctions between reality and fantasy.

A disproportionately large number of violent crimes have been carried out by Vietnam vets. It finally dawned on me that, if basically decent people with conventional moral grounding could commit such atrocities when given permission to do so, then no people have a monopoly on evil. The recent conflict in former Yugoslavia certainly illustrates this view. Thus, as a Jew, whatever lingering animosity I may have had toward Germany for what happened under the Nazi regime has vanished. Still, I strongly believe in the principle established at the Nuremberg trials, that one is ultimately responsible for his or her own actions, regardless of policies or even orders. Frankly, at the current time, anti-Arab (not antiterrorist) attitudes ("stupid", "inferior") that I have heard expressed by a few Israelis absolutely revolt me.

Just as atrocious situations can bring out the worst in people, so can they bring out the best. Some Germans hid Jews during World War II; others helped them escape (as fortunately happened to my first wife and her parents). A considerable number of American and allied soldiers performed truly heroic deeds in rescuing comrades and civilians in Vietnam. Man has the capacity for the worst (sadism) and the best (altruism) in the animal kingdom.

Incredibly, it took a decade or so after the Vietnam conflict before the establishment of "storefront" VA Vet Centers, which were intended to provide accessible ongoing psychosocial support and counseling for Vietnam vets. The person put in charge of the program was Shad Meshad, a combat vet for whom I have a great deal of respect. (In his inscription of the copy of his *Captain for Dark Mornings*, Shad wrote, "To a man who really helped validate the Vietnam veteran. I shall not forget your empathy and work in the early years when it was not popular to treat Vietnam vets.") There was agreement among those of us involved in initial planning that the centers be placed in community areas frequented by vets and not be obviously associated with VA hospitals, so as to minimize suspicion and maximize usage. I had argued for the renewal of the four-year initial authorization of funding for these centers on behalf of many vets who had not yet sought help. Regrettably, I now feel that the Vet Centers, which had become year-round hangouts for swapping war stories, had reached the point of diminishing returns and became probably no longer beneficial. Furthermore, those *still* struggling with Vietnam have serious problems that can be handled best in special VA Medical Center units for posttraumatic stress disorder or in general psychiatric units with personnel who are familiar with the syndrome.

Earlier, I made the distinction between realistic and unrealistic, or neurotic, guilt. What can one do for someone who feels guilty about having committed an atrocity? (As I said, I respect the person who is struggling with his or her conscience more than the one who is not.) In relation to war-related guilt, one could point out that reprehensible behaviors on the part of our troops were government and society authorized and, therefore, warrant *joint* responsibility. (I would sincerely say, "As an American, I, too, feel guilty about those aspects of the Vietnam War.") Insight alone, however, is not enough in dealing with realistic guilt. "Static" guilt can be converted to "animated" guilt through restitution. Self-destructiveness or self-punishment are *passive* forms of restitution. The patient must be asked how much self-destruction or unfulfillment is necessary to relieve his or her sense of guilt. Otherwise, there will be endless episodes of self-defeating behavior such as job loss, love object loss, or self-laceration.

The therapeutic alternative is *active* "symbolic" restitution. The Catholic Church offers absolution by penance. The psychiatrist can best facilitate what was recommended by St. Augustine in *Confessions*. Having been a reprobate as a young man, Augustine devoted his life to good works to the degree that he was ultimately canonized. One's harmful deeds can be used as a positive motivation to help others, counterposing what ill one has done; for example, the veteran who agonized over the torturing and killing of prostitutes in Vietnam could work at a rehabilitation center for prostitutes. Plans for symbolic restitution—actions which heal people or the environment—provide a route away from self-destructive patterns and toward life-affirming strategies.

The understanding of drug addiction and treatment arising from the Vietnam conflict will no doubt be applicable to the ever-increasing civilian problem of drug abuse among the young, many of whom share a sense of alienation from our culture in ways similar to the Vietnam vets who witnessed the horrors of a brutal, futile, and apparently meaningless war. Our inner cities are also beset by brutality, futility, and meaningless violence. A sense of purpose, significant values, and hope in the future must be reestablished.

CHAPTER IX

THE HUMAN SPIRIT IN THE LAND OF BIOLOGY

The great tragedy of life is not death but what dies within us while we live.

Norman Cousins

At about the time that I came to UCLA in 1984, Norman Cousins saw psychoneuroimmunology as a means to further his quest for proof that the patient's approach to illness brings something to bear upon the body's natural apothecary, judiciously dispensed via the brain. Although the verdict was coming in on the role of negative emotions in ill health, there was no comparable evidence that positive emotions had the opposite effect of enhancing health. Norman asked, "If the brain played an active role in the healing process, might it be consciously directed for that purpose? What would the implications of such findings be on the treatment of serious illness?" The driving force behind Norman's efforts was his belief that how the patient relates to the doctor and approaches his or her illness is essential to recovery. Norman was convinced that the UCLA Medical Center, which in recent years has consistently ranked among the top ten hospitals nationally, had at its disposal the critical mass of minds and resources necessary to establish UCLA as an international center of psychoneuroimmunology. These assets, combined with UCLA's interest in humanistic medical education, led him to join the UCLA

School of Medicine faculty in 1978 at the invitation of Dean Sherman Mellinkoff.

Norman's fascination with the potential of the human body for healing, given the right conditions provided by the physician and the patient, came about in 1964 as a result of his own recovery from a paralyzing and incurable collagen disease with a one in 500 recovery rate, known as ankylosing spondylitis. After extensive reading on collagen, he pursued a self-prescribed therapeutic regimen that included megainjections of vitamin C and laughter therapy to combat disease-aggravating emotional upheaval and, especially, to improve attitude. Norman observed that ten minutes of belly laughter would guarantee him an hour of pain-free sleep. As a professional writer, he was able to produce an eloquent and compelling account of this experience which was published in the prestigious *New England Journal of Medicine* in 1976 under the title, "Anatomy of an Illness (as Perceived by the Patient)", later to become the title of his best-selling book. His writings resulted in numerous invitations to meet with medical students and faculties nationwide and ultimately led to his appointment as Adjunct Professor of Medical Humanities at UCLA.

Two years after coming to UCLA, Norman suffered a massive heart attack. Once again, he was told that he had a dangerous and irreversible condition, to which he wryly replied, "I've heard that one before." With his physician's supervision over his regimen of diet, exercise, and stress reduction, he made a striking comeback which he documented in yet another bestseller, *The Healing Heart*. This experience fortified his belief in the resiliency of the human body. Challenged by the skepticism of many of his colleagues, he sought to document the *biological pathways* by which attitudes and emotions make their registrations on bodily systems.

As a journalist, Norman lived by the anecdote. He believed that what was true for him may well be true for others. What he needed was scientific data to support his observations, and he saw psychoneuroimmunology as the key to a new understanding of the body's, as yet not fully documented, healing system. Many mistakenly regard him as one who simply advocated laughing one's way to health.

In actuality, he used laughter as a metaphor for the full range of positive emotions (including purpose, determination, love, hope, faith, will to live, festivity) which he believed would biologically enhance the body's ability to combat disease. He never regarded the pursuit of psychological well-being as a substitute for medical treatment, but saw it as an essential way of facilitating the healing process, particularly given the fact that serious diagnoses tend to have the opposite effect of inducing panic and depression. "The fact of the matter is that serious disease requires full mobilization of resources," he wrote in a letter to the editors of *Time*, "both in terms of what medical science has to offer and the potentiation of the patient's own healing system. We do the best we can with everything within our means."

In my tribute to Norman following his death, I described his sickest patient as the *medical profession* itself, which has become overly technological and dehumanized. He set out to cure this "patient" in three ways: First, Norman tried to educate the public no longer to let themselves be treated as impersonal cases whose fate was to be determined by scanner images and laboratory data printouts. Various forms of high technology—CT and MRI scans, echocardiograms, EEG brain mapping, *ad infinitum*—have made the discerning eye, the sensitive finger, the keen ear relatively obsolete. What happened to the long and detailed (nonautomated) history-taking, the careful complete physical examination, the sensitive follow-up interviews? Economic and social forces drive medical practice. The fear of malpractice suits encourages heavy reliance on technology as a means of diagnosis. "Cost containment", however, is becoming a worse villain than technology as patients are processed in assembly line fashion and fewer, as well as shorter, physician visits become required by non-physician-led medical organizations. "Informed consent" forms, listing every possible complication and adverse outcome, mainly for the legal protection of the physician, can instill fear and pessimism in patients. Time spent talking to patients is not paid for. Norman encouraged patients to insist upon such "cognitive services". (A few years ago, as Chair of its Committee on Mental Health, I persuaded the California Medical Association to join forces with the Society for General Internal Medicine in an attempt to obtain legally mandated reimbursement for cognitive services. They failed.) Cost-effectiveness of such physician-patient relationship issues should now be subjected to proof by direct research, as psychoneuroimmunologic evidence so suggests. Norman urged patients to begin demanding appropriate compensation for physicians who attend to their dietary habits and work pressures in order to obviate the need for, say, a $10,000 coronary angioplasty.

Second, Norman tried to change the way that medical students are taught. He was instrumental in the development of courses on "doctoring" at UCLA Medical School that addressed the importance of patient-physician communication and the patient's involvement in his or her own treatment program. Norman would remind medical students in graduation speeches that, "There are qualities beyond pure medical competence that patients need and look for in doctors . . . They want to be looked after and not just looked over . . . Ultimately, it is the physician's respect for the human soul that determines the worth of his science." He even noted that it was in the physician's self-interest to develop a good rapport with the patient. Doctors often have to be master psychologists in eliciting information and in developing attitudes and behaviors in patients that promote effective treatment. Norman also felt strongly that a good patient-physician relationship would dramatically reduce the risk of malpractice suits. In his mailbox survey of residents in Westwood, the community nearest the UCLA campus, he found that 85 percent of respondents had changed physicians within the past five years, most citing the style or personality of the physician as the reason for changing doctors. (Unfortunately, more and more systems of medical care delivery do not permit choice of physicians.)

Perhaps in the future, premedical studies in the humanities, social sciences, and even economics will turn out to be as relevant to medical practice as chemistry and physics. Perhaps medical students of the future will be chosen not only for their test-taking abilities in quantitative subjects but also for their humanistic characteristics, their ability to reason, and their original thought. Not long ago, I observed a medical student taking a patient's history. During the "Review of Systems", the student asked, "Any problems with your eyes?" The patient suffering from cancer replied, "They water because I am sad." Another question promptly ensued, "Any pus?" Would a medical school course in psychoneuroimmunology help that student understand that sadness might be relevant to cancer prognosis? Modeling is more effective than teaching *per se*. Recall my experiences in London as a medical student. Professor McMichael, himself a contributor to high-tech medicine, never would have been so callous! Students no longer "stand at the elbows" of the likes of a McMichael.

Third, Norman tried to establish the scientific basis for humanistic medicine by encouraging research in the field of psychoneuroimmunology, particularly research that dared to place the human spirit in the land of biology. Data can do that. Will "left-brained", nonintuitive, evidence-oriented physicians then become more humane? Maybe. Norman envisioned a program that would not only produce sophisticated research in the field but also set the standards for the development of an integrative approach to health and disease, one that would acknowledge the psychological profile of the patient as a fundamental part of diagnosis and treatment and, correspondingly, recognize the importance of communication with and empathy for patients in creating an auspicious environment for treatment.

In pursuit of this dream, Norman held extensive discussions with Dean Sherman Mellinkoff, Jolly West, Franklin Murphy (physician and former Chancellor of UCLA), and Carmine Clemente (Director of the Brain Research Institute). Their consensus was that Norman should create a psychoneuroimmunology task force of high-caliber scientists, whose representation encompassed the breadth of relevant disciplines, to serve as a think tank appraising PNI and strategizing its development at UCLA. He did so, and out of the task force grew the UCLA Program in Psychoneuroimmunology, dedicated to the promotion of excellence in the field. Norman particularly encouraged the funding of first-of-its-kind human research. Although he believed in the importance of funding molecular research, he kept the group from getting lost in the molecules (a danger even to PNI, which

some prefer to call "neuroimmunomodulation") by continually remind-
ing that all medical research should be aimed at alleviating human
suffering. With these goals in mind, the program provides "seed"
grants to UCLA faculty, reaching beyond the "already converted" by
encouraging molecular scientists to add psychological components to
their research and, conversely, by inviting behavioral scientists to add
biological components to their work. The research program gets a
major boost from its state-of-the-art Psychoneuroimmunology Core
Laboratory, directed by John Fahey, which services the entire campus
and is devoted to psychoneuroimmunologic research (with free services available to postdoctoral fellows in PNI).

The educational component of the program targets everyone, from
community members to UCLA faculty. A clinical clerkship in PNI,
organized by Fawzy Fawzy, is offered for medical students from UCLA
and elsewhere. The centerpiece of psychoneuroimmunologic education at UCLA is the postdoctoral training program. This program
immerses trainees in disciplines radically different from their original
areas of expertise. This truly interdisciplinary training produces individuals capable of *thinking* in multiple biobehavioral "languages"
(rather than merely possessing a rudimentary knowledge of them).
From this ability to integrate disparate frames of reference comes the
potential for developing genuine breakthroughs. The postdoctoral
training program accepts applicants from all over the world (since it
does not depend upon U.S. government training grants) and then sends
them back into the world in order to spawn the international development of first-rate, health relevant, psychoneuroimmunologic work.
A visiting lecturer series and periodic cutting-edge conferences serve
to inform the community, promote networking, and elevate the quality and health relevance of research. For example, a recent conference
was held on the application of nonlinear dynamics (the mathematics
of chaos) to medicine, with all its complex interactions of multiple
feedback loops, especially psycho-neuro-endocrine-immune.

There were two "angels" who made all of this possible. Just prior to
the establishment of the PNI Task Force, Mrs. Joan Kroc (widow of
Ray Kroc, founder of the McDonald's chain of fast-food restaurants)

requested a meeting with Norman. They met at a hotel restaurant in La Jolla, where he learned of her foundation dedicated to the remediation of the human condition, particularly substance abuse. He was struck by how well-informed and socially concerned she was. Mrs. Kroc told Norman that she was familiar with his work and, believing that his objectives had useful implications for health and medical treatment, offered him $2,000,000 with which he could promote research documenting the value of positive emotions for health. At Norman's urging, Mrs. Kroc attended the first meetings of the task force, flying in from home near San Diego on her helicopter and landing on the hospital emergency rooftop landing pad. A few years later, after the original $2,000,000 had been spent but an additional $5,000,000 had been accrued, the remarkable Mrs. Kroc advised Norman to use the money in a self-sustaining endowment fashion, spending only the interest from the invested capital. Pleased by its progress and solid in her commitment, she assisted the program in meeting its annual budgetary needs by bolstering the endowment with an additional $3,000,000. Mrs. Kroc recognized that progress only comes from taking risks; she had the courage and conviction to do so. In my few contacts with Joan Kroc, I was truly impressed by her compassion (as exemplified by the Ronald McDonald houses for families of children with life-threatening illnesses), genuineness, and generosity. Would that all persons of comparable means were like her!

The other $5,000,000 had come from another angel, Mrs. Burton Bettingen. She had been named after her father, Burton Green, the developer of Beverly Hills who had wisely invested his profits in Bakersfield oil, leaving his three daughters enormously wealthy. Mrs. Bettingen was a benefactor of UCLA, whose previously exciting and meaningful life had deteriorated with her health. She called Dean Mellinkoff to ask if Norman might speak to her. (Norman gave hope and encouragement to hundreds of patients each year, never charging a dime for his services.) Through a series of visits over a period of six weeks, she regained her sense of purpose by discovering that she could still make a difference in the world through anonymous giving. In gratitude, she sent the Dean a check for $50,000 to be used at

Norman's discretion. The next time Norman saw her, Mrs. Bettingen asked what he had done with the check. He replied, "Nothing. I put it away in an account." Upon further interrogation, he explained that he would be putting it toward the development of a Program in Psychoneuroimmunology. After briefly describing the program's goals and research achievements as a result of Mrs. Kroc's original gift, Mrs. Bettingen asked, "Do you have any idea what a permanent program would cost?" Recalling one of his advisors giving an off-the-top-of-his-head estimate of $5,000,000 he said, "$5 million." She wrote him a check for $4,950,000, but asked him to wait a day before cashing it because she had bought some lingerie the day before and wanted to be sure that there was enough money in the account. Subsequently, Mrs. Bettingen wrote yet another check for $5,000,000 with the request that Norman return for it, again because she needed to transfer money into her checking account, but she died of a heart attack that very night before the transaction was completed. At first, her executors intended to honor her wishes, particularly since she had had unquestionably full mental capacity prior to her death; however, they reneged. Although it likely could have won, the university appropriately did not wish to engender bad publicity and ill will in filing suit against the estate, as had been Norman's first impulse.

Norman was a man of mission. "My dedication, therefore, is to the cause of man in the attainment of that which is within the reach of man." As its 30-year editor, Norman used the *Saturday Review* as a forum to pique the conscience of its readers. His editorials called for reform in areas such as unsafe medical practices, educational standards, pollution control, violent entertainment, cigarette advertising, and military intervention in third world countries. He was particularly committed to exploring the implications of the Atomic Age. As a result of the emergence of weapons capable of mass destruction, he argued passionately that the world was now engaged in a common struggle for survival; individual nations could no longer afford to commit unmitigated acts of aggression on their neighbors. "Nothing is more powerful," he affirmed, "than an individual acting out of his conscience, thus helping to bring the collective conscience to life."

Although Norman dealt in global matters, he never lost sight of individual suffering. He rallied support from his *Saturday Review* readership to provide for the care and education of 400 children orphaned as a result of the atomic explosion in Hiroshima and for a surgical reconstruction program for 25 young, severely disfigured Japanese women (called the "Hiroshima maidens").

Not surprisingly, Norman had gigantic plans for the Program in Psychoneuroimmunology. Prior to his death, he had been well on his way toward getting commitments for $50,000,000 to expand it into a major center for the field. Probably as a vestige of his diplomatic work, Norman played his cards close to his vest. Other than potential donors, the only people who knew about his plans were the Dean of the Medical School, myself, and the leaders of the two outstanding groups in psychoneuroimmunology whom he had hoped to attract to UCLA—Ronald Glaser and Janice Kiecolt-Glaser of Ohio State University; and experimental psychologist Robert Ader, neurophysiologist David Felten, and immunologist Nicholas Cohen of the University of Rochester. Had Norman lived only a brief time longer, the center would have materialized.

Norman died in an enviable but untimely manner, having gone to the luxurious Westwood Marquis Hotel for afternoon tea, where he collapsed with a heart attack. Of course, sudden death, while easier on Norman, was very hard on those dear to him. Norman led an active and full life to the very end. In the years prior to his death he wrote several books, two of which I liked in particular: *The Human Adventure* (a chronicle of his own photographs) and *The Pathology of Power* (an analysis of the dangers inherent in a military-industrial complex). Norman actually survived for a decade after his cardiologist had said that he was at grave risk for dying within a year were he not to have coronary bypass surgery, which he had refused. Would he have lived long enough to see the center materialize if he had had the bypass surgery? He may have, but more important to him was the opportunity to demonstrate human potential. Maybe I should have been suspicious of his impending death because Norman, usually a patient man, seemed to have a sense of urgency about the development of the center in the weeks prior to his death. He was extremely tuned in to his own bodily processes; perhaps he sensed something awry. Some who worked closely with him speculate that he knew he was not well during the last month of his life and that he chose to leave this world with a bang, not a whimper. After his death, the program was re-named The Norman Cousins Program in Psychoneuroimmunology at UCLA.

After dinner at Norman's home above Beverly Hills, he would lead a discussion almost in the style of a 19th century salon. One evening after hearing an elegant commentary on the nature of the modern theater by the renowned, elderly drama coach, the late Stella Adler (one of the founders of the Method school of acting and teacher of Marlon Brando, among others), Norman, to my surprise and alarm, asked me to talk about psychoneuroimmunology and AIDS. I quickly thought, "What in the world does psychoneuroimmunology have to do with Method acting?" Perhaps Norman was prescient. It was not much later that psychology graduate student Ann Futterman (who went on to join the faculty of the University of Colorado), with sup-port provided by the PNI Task Force, demonstrated that professional method actors had lowered immunity after reenacting despair. Con-versely, states of elation were followed by enhanced T cell immunity, as measured by lymphocyte responsiveness to mitogen. Norman was always eager to experiment on himself. Once, after participating in a session with a group of long-survivors of AIDS that I had assembled, he had his blood drawn by Dan Stites at the UCSF Clinical Immu-nology Laboratory for lymphocyte subset analysis before and after a brief period of intense, positive thought. "That should enhance my immunity!" (It did, at least in terms of numbers of cytotoxic cells.) Years later, I asked what he had been thinking about, and Norman replied, "World peace and nuclear disarmament."

A recent leap for the field has been the establishment of an en-dowed Norman Cousins Chair in Psychoneuroimmunology at UCLA, the first PNI Chair in the United States. (There is one in The Neth-erlands.) Without saying anything to anyone at UCLA, including other members of the Psychoneuroimmunology Task Force, Ellen

(Eleanor) Cousins and I flew off to Kalamazoo, Michigan, to ask the leadership of the Fetzer Institute for the endowment. (Ellen, Norman's widow, with whom Susan and I have remained close, is an expert in nutrition and a remarkable person in her own right,) Kalamazoo is home to the magnificent headquarters of the Fetzer Institute, founded by inventor and broadcast entrepreneur John Fetzer, that is devoted to the study of the integration of mind, body, and spirit. I had always felt that psychoneuroimmunology was just "up its alley", as had Bob Ader who was on their Advisory Board. Fetzer's foresighted President, Robert Lehman, arranged for the Institute's largest gift ever—$1 million to UCLA to establish the Norman Cousins Chair. Ellen and I were thrilled, as was everyone at UCLA.

Beyond my interest in PNI and aging, I remained committed to the study of the psychoneuroimmunologic aspects of HIV/AIDS, some of which has already been described. This interest was facilitated by the presence of UCLA's Margaret Kemeny, whom I had first met while she was a postdoctoral fellow in health psychology at UCSF. Margaret eventually joined and then headed the Psychoneuroimmunology Task Force at UCLA. She obtained a sizable grant to investigate psychological correlates of HIV progression, as measured by biological markers. Margaret's prospective study involved the ongoing evaluation of a group of about 1,000 gay and bisexual men enrolled in the Los Angeles MACS, the previously described long-term study documenting the natural evolution of HIV infection. The subjects were very similar to those we had studied at the UCSF Biopsychosocial AIDS Project, and a number of Margaret's findings complemented our earlier findings. Following bereavement, HIV seropositive gay men show a significant rise in detrimental immune activation as well as a decrease in the ability of their T cells to respond to mitogen. A poorly done study from another institution claimed that depression was not related to the progression of disease in asymptomatic HIV positive men. That study had only measured depression at one point in time and followed up on health status six months later without determining whether or not the subjects were still depressed. Margaret's research team found, rather, that individuals suffering from sustained depressed mood (high depression on five of six ratings over a two-year period) had an 80% chance of experiencing a steep decline in helper T cell numbers compared to a 30% chance of that type of decline in persons who were not continuously "bummed out". They also noted that "fatalism", or a sense of powerlessness over the virus (probably better described as "pessimism"), predicted a steep decline in helper T cell numbers and, thus, progression to AIDS and death.

Immunologic defects in HIV, which are predictive of disease progression, include not only depletion of CD4 cells but also inappropriate activation of components of the immune system. Evidence of unnecessary activation includes: elevations in the number of activation markers (such as CD25) on the surface of T cells; increases in beta-2 microglobulin and neopterin (the latter produced by macrophages); and overproduction of immunoglobulins (antibodies) that are not specific for any microorganism (a polyclonal expansion by B cells). "Overtaxed" B cells are less able to respond to specific new invaders. Now the "gold standard" for assessment of disease progression, drug efficacy, and patient prognosis is the measure of actual numbers of human immunodeficiency virus particles (virions) in the blood, made possible by the perfection of new technology. We are using these "viral load" tests in our new psychoneuroimmunologic research in HIV/AIDS.

Although HIV invades cells possessing the CD4 receptor, direct invasion by virus does not account for all the CD4 T cells that are lost. Autoimmunity may be one explanation, since lymphocytes not actually invaded by virus that have gp120 (a soluble viral protein that has floated off the surface of HIV) stuck on their surface may be recognized as foreign and killed by other lymphocytes. A different mechanism whereby uninfected CD4 cells become depleted may be via increased apoptosis, or accelerated programmed cell death, perhaps also induced by gp120. If autoimmunity is a factor in HIV progression, are Rudy Moos's and my findings regarding psychological factors in autoimmune diseases relevant?

One of Margaret's gifted postdoctoral students, Christian Hart, on whose dissertation committee I served, found that vivid negative imagery regarding the outcome of one's own disease was associated with a lower proliferative response of T cells to mitogen in HIV positive men. Unfortunately, Chris was unable to validate his hypothesis that strong positive images would be associated with better prognosis and that less vivid imagery of any sort would have correspondingly less prognostic significance. Perhaps his longitudinal follow-up of the original cross-sectional study may prove the hypothesis that strong imagery has self-fulfilling potential. Unlike Freud's view of mental health as being represented by good reality testing, UCLA psychologist Shelley Taylor defines mental health as seeing the world through "rose colored glasses", or having a more positive—even "unrealistic"—view of the future. In her book, *Positive Illusions*, she asserts that much of life is the result of anticipation and self-fulfilling prophecy; for example, if an average-looking young woman considers herself unattractive, she is less likely to go out on dates or get married than a similar-looking woman who considers herself attractive and behaves as if she were desirable and good-looking. Both Shelley and I, as did Norman Cousins, believe that one's psychological outlook colors the course of *physical* as well as mental health. (Realistic appraisal of situations, however, may at times also promote good health, which I discovered in a study of earthquake victims described later.)

In a nine-year prospective study following gay and bisexual men, Steven Cole (another highly gifted, postdoctoral fellow co-mentored by Margaret and me) found that HIV positive gay men "in the closet", who hide their sexual orientation from family and coworkers (even though they may reveal it to some other gay people), proceed to AIDS-defining illness and death *one-and-a-half to two years* sooner than men who are open about their sexuality. While lecturing in Colombia, I pointed out that the prejudicial Latin attitude against homosexuality that forces gay people to hide their sexuality actually has major negative public health implications. For instance, a Chilean psychiatrist friend and colleague, who had been trained in the United States, told me that a prominent friend of his was HIV positive and asked if I would speak to him about my research. I asked if the friend was gay; he didn't know, but assumed not. Having put the friend at ease with openness about my own sexuality, I found out that he was indeed gay but had not even told his best friend (my colleague). I urged him to do so, to give himself at least one person in whom he could confide. For fear of being discovered, he had avoided having sexual relations in Chile, seeking them in foreign centers like Rio instead.

Still intrigued by the exception to the rule, I began to look more systematically at a very rare group of individuals: those with HIV who had never been symptomatic or who had been asymptomatic for over six months after a single bout of an AIDS-defining illness during which time their CD4 cell counts had remained below a 50 per cubic millimeter. The newer definition of AIDS as a CD4 cell number below $200/mm^3$ by the Centers for Disease Control, I believe, is psychologically detrimental. Disease should be defined *clinically*. Being labeled as having AIDS while still well can be depressing and likely can accelerate the appearance of clinical disease. By the time CD4 cell counts get below 50, AIDS-defining symptoms such as wasting syndrome, AIDS dementia complex, and opportunistic infections are generally present. (Kaposi's Sarcoma can occur at counts somewhat above 200.) An ongoing study of HIV positive asymptomatic persons in San Francisco has documented that 87% of those with CD4 cell counts of less than 200 at entry progressed to AIDS within three years. Only 25% of HIV positive men who did not develop an AIDS-defining illness over the course of ten years had counts below 200; undoubtedly, far fewer had levels below 50. It is not clear what biological factors could account for well-being with so few CD4 cells. As I said, I had postulated that natural killer (NK) cells, which have been shown in many studies to be sensitive to both depression and other forms of psychological distress, might be the compensatory mechanism in persons who remain asymptomatic in spite of so *few* CD4 cells. New work, both completed and in progress at UCLA, on long-survivors and relatively healthy individuals with very low CD4 cell counts was described in Chapter IV.

There is another group of unusual HIV-infected individuals that I have wanted to study: the 5-10% of the HIV positive population that not only have remained asymptomatic for 10+ years but also have not shown significant declines in their CD4 cells, remaining in the near-normal to normal range of CD4 cell counts (500-800), so-called "nonprogressors." Even mild AIDS-related symptoms do not tend to occur until CD4 cell counts fall below 500, so these are essentially healthy HIV-infected individuals. What might keep the disease from progressing? There are three possibilities: genetics, weak virus, or good immunity. That genetics are involved is suggested by the fact that some highly exposed individuals never get infected in the first place. It has been discovered that these people lack a second receptor (CCR5) that is now known to have to be present besides the CD4 receptor for HIV to enter the cell. Could a partial absence of CCR5 lead to partial resistance (nonprogression)?

Unlike herpes simplex virus, HIV is not a latent virus. Although there may be very low levels of virus in the bloodstream, a lymph node biopsy will reveal a large amount of virus. With the continual replication of virus in the lymph nodes, a person whose disease has not progressed must be able to kill several billion viral particles a day as well as replace killed cells. [UCLA immunologist Janis Giorgi and others postulated that a particular type of cytotoxic T cell (CD8+CD38-HLA-DR+) may be responsible for producing a substance (chemokine) that can attack HIV.] Such a feat requires a prodigiously powerful immune system, particularly in light of HIV's propensity for mutation into different forms. As mentioned earlier, the ever-changing nature of the virus leads to the development of resistance to antiretroviral drugs. A major advance in the use of protease inhibitor drugs, was the realization that to prevent or delay viral resistance they had to be used in simultaneous combination with two or three reverse transcriptase inhibitor drugs. The newer protease inhibitor drugs inhibit a different enzyme (protease) that is involved in "cutting" the virus to the correct, virulent length. The precisely-timed consumption of multiple expensive pills comprising protease/reverse transcriptase inhibitor "cocktails" must be continued indefinitely, lest viral load quickly resurge. Although combinations of drugs represent a significant advance, real progress against disease awaits new medications or methods. Molecular biological approaches are promising. So far, there are only a few documented cases of recovery from HIV infection, those of children who had both HIV and antibodies to the virus in their blood at birth, but who, by two to four years of age, no longer had any trace of the antibodies or the virus. Apart from the relative efficacy of various drugs with varied toxicities (side-effects), and the vicissitudes of viral "virulence" and mutation, there remains—as in other infectious diseases—the issue of *host resistance (immunologic)* to the virus. (This topic was—at last—emphasized in the International Congress on AIDS held in Vancouver, B.C. in 1996.) Such immunologic resistance as I already have tried convincingly to show, is affected by psychological factors. Thus, I strongly suspect that the biological health of nonprogressors is accompanied by an equally remarkable psychological fortitude, partial resistance. We are now conducting psychological evaluations of nonprogressing research subjects in a manner similar to our study of long-survivors. Perhaps CD8+CD38-HLA-DR+ cells are psychologically sensitive! The continuing absence of truly curative medical treatments makes psychoneuroimmunologic approaches all the more important.

In 1986, I came down with herpes zoster ("shingles"). Herpes zoster is caused by varicella virus that also causes chicken pox. The virus lies dormant in peripheral nerves for a lifetime. Like other herpes group viruses, its activation is especially likely to occur under conditions of stress, aging, or HIV, which suppress cellular immune defenses. I had had chicken pox at age three and a bout with zoster followed by several months of postherpetic intercostal (between the ribs) pain when I was 25 years old, during my somewhat stressful first year of psychiatric residency. Therefore, I was not particularly concerned. Although I was taking oral doses of an effective antiherpes virus drug, acyclovir, the zoster affected my right trigeminal (facial sensory) nerve at an alarming rate of progression. (Thankfully, it did not affect the ophthalmic branch, which can lead to blindness.) My face swelled enormously; I looked like a monster. I had never been so ill with such high fevers and had to be hospitalized for nearly a week (deliberately not at UCLA) in order to receive massive intravenous doses of acyclovir. At that time, it was erroneously thought that herpes zoster in an HIV positive person meant the development of full-blown AIDS within one or two years. I requested HIV antibody testing. I was positive.

A good portion of the terror subsided when testing revealed that my wife and former lover (now happily remarried and still a close friend) had tested negative. I asked my good friend Michael Gottlieb (who, recall, named AIDS in 1981) to be my doctor. He still is. I told my brother and sons. Toward the end of that year, I uncharacteristically decided to throw a big party for my 55th birthday, asking my brother Daniel to come from San Francisco, figuring it might be my last. Also a former Stanford undergraduate, Dan gave me a Stanford football jersey with the number 55 on the back. (Daniel is Professor of Architecture at the University of California, Berkeley, a renowned residential architect and urban planner.)

Fourteen years later, my CD4 cell count is over 800 (normal) My viral load is "undetectable" by standard techniques and very, very low by special supersensitive methodology. Clearly, I am a nonprogressor.

My initial infection likely occurred about 20 years ago. Dr. Gottlieb tells me that I shall not die of AIDS, rather of chronic lung disease secondary to nearly lifelong asthma. (Psychodynamically, is having a severe allergic disease why I became interested in psychological-immune connections in the first place?) Mike even talked me into taking anticholesterol medication lest I have a heart attack! Except for not having the stamina that I did 30 years ago, I have had no serious illnesses in the last decade, and I feel just fine. I work hard, ski, and play tennis, just as I have always done. Why have I been self-revealing? Well, I am an interesting case! Importantly, I admire courage and forthrightness. Perhaps, I can set an example.

On the other hand, maybe I'm a fool since the Gay and Lesbian Medical Association strongly advises nonrevelation. Many of its HIV positive members are without jobs despite the fact that there has not been a single report of doctor to patient transmission other than one possible instance in France and the inexplicable situation of the Florida dentist, Dr. Acer, that led to widespread panic and some bad policy decisions.

Am I just lucky to have a relatively benign strain of virus or a genetically adaptive immune system, or do my psychological characteristics and social supports, as might be inferred by the reader, play a role in my inclusion among the five to 10 percent of persons whose disease does not seem to progress? (Of course, there is still the possibility that my CD4 cells could "crash".) Luc Montagnier had told me that he thought, barring development of effective treatment for HIV (God forbid), in 5,000 years or so HIV would cause a rather benign disease, just as SIV (simian immunodeficiency virus) does in African monkeys. Monkeys from Asia, where SIV is not endemic, die within one or two years after inoculation with the virus. A certain small percentage of the population of a species, he believes, has natural immunity to any microorganism. Then, survival of the fittest prevails. Thus, perhaps I'm just lucky with my genes. Older HIV positive persons may actually have a worse prognosis because of age-related declines in immune function. I have no formula for nonprogression. I carry on life as usual without worrying about illness and try to find meaning in life. I take vitamins, exercise, and [not enough] vacations. (Fourteen years ago, Susan and I splurged on what we thought was an idyllic "last" vacation on Turtle Island, Fiji.) I'm not depressed. (Obviously, were I young and not yet fulfilled, this might not be the case.) Shakespeare had it right (*Julius Caesar*):

> *Cowards die many times before their deaths.*
> *The valiant never taste of death but once.*
> *Of all the wonders that I yet have heard,*
> *It seems to me most strange that men should fear,*
> *Seeing that death, a necessary end,*
> *Will come when it will come.*

Life has been anything but stress-free. In the past few years, my home was damaged by earthquake, fire, and flood. In pages to follow, I shall describe the toll that the Northridge earthquake, in destroying my office and labs, has taken on my career as well. I cope. In virtually any situation, I can find something interesting or instructive, or funny. I don't characteristically hold back in expressing my feelings, unless I suspect that I am off-base. I most value contributing to human knowledge, helping others, being socially responsible, being a good friend, father, and husband (and having sports cars). I am convinced that my ability to cope plays a significant role in my health. I tell all this in the hope that other HIV seropositive persons may benefit and, thus, at least in my opinion, live healthily longer.

My life changed on January 17, 1994, the day of the Northridge earthquake. The Sepulveda VA Medical Center and its campus consisting of about a dozen buildings is located about a mile from the epicenter of the earthquake. Built in the 1950s, its main building containing medical and surgical units had seams that pulled apart, saving the building from complete collapse; however, with the failure of the main backup power system for the entire campus, as well as the failure of four backup systems in the main building, all patients on life support died (something not reported in the casualty figures). The staff on duty behaved heroically, dragging sick patients on mattresses across gaps in the floor and down stairwells in the dark. Many of us could not get to the hospital because of damage to our homes or the freeways. My office was very badly damaged; 2,500 books lay on the floor like shuffled cards. All laboratories had to be decontaminated because of broken glassware containing toxic chemicals and radioactive materials. With the help of more auxiliary generators, a temporary boiler for hot water, and cellular phones, we endeavored to maintain outpatient services using outdoor areas as needed. It was a terrible mess. In addition, there was great uncertainty as to whether the Federal Government would rebuild the facility through its Department of Veterans Affairs; after all, UCLA still had affiliation with another VA hospital adjacent to campus, West Los Angeles VA Medical Center. (The Sepulveda staff, including me, liked to think of itself as the better of the two.)

I felt that these highly stressful, acute circumstances presented an ideal opportunity for research on the psychoneuroimmunologic effects of a natural disaster. Lydia Temoshok had tried to do a similar study at UCSF after the Loma Prieta quake in the San Francisco Bay Area, but the "fast track" $50,000 funding from NIMH arrived three months too late. She returned the money. A bit of earthquake data had been gathered on October 1, 1987, when Margaret Kemeny had drawn blood on her laboratory personnel at UCLA one to two hours following a relatively minor quake (magnitude 5.4 as opposed to 6.7 in Northridge). She found no changes in T cell activity, but did find increases in NK cell activity, as one would expect in response to acute stress. With enormous cooperation from members of the Research and Education Committee at the Sepulveda VA Medical Center, whose own lives had been highly disrupted, I obtained approval for my frantically written proposal to study psychological and immunologic sequelae of the Northridge quake, using employees of the VA hospital as subjects. I was greatly aided in this work by the previously-mentioned Viennese physician in postdoctoral training, Peter Grohr, who with his lively and disarming interpersonal skills was able to elicit cooperation from the badly shaken up (literally as well as figuratively) employees for the blood draws and psychological tests. He even chased down employees who had followed their patients to other VA institutions. Just before the second round of blood drawing, the Secretary of Veterans Affairs Jessie Brown flew out from Washington, D.C., to announce (in a large, hastily-erected tent) that because of the enormous cost of reconstruction and the existing duplication of facilities with West Los Angeles, the full hospital would not be rebuilt. The hospital would be transformed into a much smaller "state-of-the-art" outpatient facility, since a pilot ambulatory care center had already been begun using teams of physicians, including psychiatrists (an excellent model for modern, lower cost, integrated medical care). Many staff would be transferred to other VA facilities around the country or encouraged to retire. Most researchers began to seek opportunities elsewhere.

In our earthquake study, we had the unique opportunity to compare subjective ratings of psychological distress with objective measures of life disruption: whether or not the employee's unit was still functioning or threatened with possible closure, whether or not the person's job was at stake, how much damage there was to the individual's home, whether or not the employee had earthquake insurance, whether or not the person's ability to get to work was severely impaired by road damage, and whether or not injuries or death had occurred to friends or family (as turned out to be the case for 60% of the employees in our study). Over the course of four months, we found that the degree of emotional distress decreased to about half its initial level; however, T cell function and natural killer cell cytotoxic activity continued to decline in a linear manner. Thus, *duration*, and not just intensity of stress, is relevant to immune function. An even more fascinating finding, unique to this study, was that CD8 cells were more negatively impacted by a subjective emotional response that was disproportionate to the actual amount of life disruption. In other words, people whose houses had been destroyed, whose jobs were at risk, and who had injured family members but who downplayed the impact and admitted little distress ("Well, its just one of those things", "That's the way life goes") had *more* immunosuppression than those who were more grossly distressed ("Oh, my God, this is one of the worst things that ever happened to me", "What am I going to do?", "I'm terribly worried"). Similarly, those whose workplace was still functioning and whose homes had relatively little damage, yet who were terribly freaked out showed *more* immune dysfunction than those whose reactions were proportional to the event. We were unable to measure the reactions of those who experienced the greatest degree of panic. They fled the area immediately after the quake or had not yet returned to work at the commencement of blood drawing. For instance, my gracious, "aging Southern belle" secretary, only after receiving a tranquilizer prescription from me over the telephone, managed to take the first available flight out to Kentucky; she had to be carried off the plane in a stretcher. My paper, "Shaking Up Immunity", ensued. Gail Ironson has studied victims of Hurricane Andrew, who had had some warning before the disaster and, therefore, some advantage in their ability to cope. I suggested that she title her paper, "Blowing Out Immunity". (She was chicken and didn't.) Gail's much longer follow-up (4 years) showed that NK cell function remained lower in those who continued to have intrusive thoughts of the disaster (posttraumatic stress disorder). In a comparison of the psychological sequelae of the two disasters, graduate student Suzanne Segerstrom (now on the faculty of the University of Kentucky), Gail, and I found that, while degree of damage to home and possessions was correlated with trauma-related distress in both disasters, the earthquake was associated with more fear of death and more intrusively experienced thoughts, feelings, and nightmares.

Most of my colleagues at Sepulveda, including Bruce Naliboff, opted for transfer to the West Los Angeles VA Medical Center. However, I decided to take the modest early retirement package offered by the VA and return to the UCLA campus, where I was able to continue my research with support of the Psychoneuroimmunology Task Force under the aegis of Carmine Clemente. When Norman died, the leadership of the task force was left in the hands of Carmine, an experienced administrator and top flight anatomist. Carmine, editor of the major anatomy text and atlas, had headed the Brain Research Institute at UCLA until political infighting forced him from the position. He has never done any research in psychoneuroimmunology. Presumably, Norman had named him successor (that very issue being rather unclear after Norman's sudden death) by virtue of his administrative skills and good connections within the medical school. Norman had been a benevolent despot, running the program by himself (albeit with good input from the task force on actual research projects and selection of postdoctoral fellows). To the disgruntlement of the task force members, Carmine continued to handle matters in the same manner as Norman had, even though the funds had explicitly been given to the university to be used at Norman's discretion and not at the discretion of his successor. Carmine eventually stepped aside, and was replaced on an interim basis by my old friend Margaret Kemeny. She will be replaced by whomever is chosen as the Norman Cousins Professor. Carmine's legitimate, but unfortunately limited, goal had been to balance the program's budget. Not one penny had been added to the PNI endowment at UCLA during Carmine's reign.

Fortunately, Margaret has played a central role in focusing the program's research effort on two areas which have always been of

great interest to me, autoimmune/inflammatory diseases and mechanisms of alternative healing. By good fortune, I was called by Janet
Stein, wife of the founder of the Dreyfus Funds, who has a particular
interest in Ayurveda, which I had gone to India to learn about so
many years ago. She promptly sent me a check (of course, made out
to the University of California Regents) for $30,000. Supplemented
to $100,000, it supported a psychoneuroimmunologic study of the ef-
fects of meditation on the clinical course and immunology of inflammatory bowel disease.

Since I was neither receiving university salary nor requiring my
active professor status in order to continue teaching and research, I
elected to assume emeritus status, which carried with it all the privileges of a full professorship minus the political pressures, administrative headaches, bureaucratic hassles, and mandatory teaching load.
Although I had been initially provided neither the salary nor the
space that I had wished from the university, they were predictably
forthcoming after my receipt of the unexpected $1.6 million AIDS
long-survivor grant (split with the University of Miami). The University takes 49% of that money as overhead, but does not even pay for
the telephone!

For many years, I routinely declined opportunities to testify in
civil cases involving physical illness following mental distress resulting from negligence or malfeasance. I had felt that there was already
a vast overexaggeration of claims in the courts for mental stress *per se*
and for worker's compensation based on stress rather than injury.
Mounting evidence of the adverse effects of severe stressors on immunity and health, however, have led me to testify in a *few* select
cases, particularly involving infectious diseases that are clearly resisted by immunity. Immune resistance to cancer is less clear-cut and
can depend on the type of tumor. The role of the immune system in
cancer is best demonstrated in non-Hodgkin's lymphoma (a manifesta-
tion of AIDS) and malignant melanoma, for which augmentation of
specific immunity can sometimes have dramatic therapeutic effects.

I testified on behalf of an emotionally stable, high-achieving,
athletic UCLA student (Randall) whose Volkswagen convertible, which
he had spent many hours and $15,000 to restore, was destroyed when

he was rear-ended at a stop light by a truck with defective brakes. At the UCLA emergency room, Randall was found to have no internal injuries or fractures, only bruises and muscle strains. X-rays were all negative. Nonetheless, he was in considerable physical discomfort and emotional distress. For his beloved car, the insurance company would only pay $3,000—its unrestored value. Randall was unable to study for or take his finals, causing him to lose a quarter's (three months) worth of academic credit. Moreover, he had no means of transportation from his apartment to the university. Three days following the accident, Randall suddenly developed severe abdominal pain. He was found to have peritonitis (infection of the membrane that lines the walls of the abdominal cavity), an abscess under his diaphragm near the spleen, and septicemia (a life-endangering condition in which pathogenic microorganisms permeate the bloodstream). The spleen was removed, and he was hospitalized for over two months. When Randall recovered, he was forced to give up his treasured independence to live with his parents, his father being a loving but rather authoritarian former military officer. Three months later, he had another episode of peritonitis, requiring further surgery to drain pus from the abdomen and several more weeks of hospitalization. Six months later, Randall suffered from intestinal obstruction caused by scarring from the prior inflammation (adhesions) and had to undergo *another* laparotomy. Why did this young man of prior good health develop a massive bacterial infection without any apparent source? The temporal relationship between the accident and the onset of a rare and massive bacterial infection strongly suggested distress-related immunosuppression as a contributing factor. After my deposition the insurance company settled for a considerable sum, not wanting the case to go to trial lest even more money be awarded by a sympathetic jury. Although my conservatism in drawing conclusions makes me a more credible witness, I still worry about contributing to an increasingly litigious society. On the one hand, it seems fair to reimburse for culpable behaviors. On the other hand, in the U.S. legal system in which the plaintiff's attorney can be guaranteed a contingency fee equal to 40% of the settlement plus expenses, and the plaintiff is not required to fork out a cent, there is high potential for abuse. Will psychoneuroimmunology open a "Pandora's box" of already extensive stress-related litigation?

I do not want the narrative of this professional saga to end on an academic, political, or forensic note but, rather, on a *clinical* one. Professionally, I feel that I am a DOCTOR above all. Therefore, sadly, I shall recount a recent patient of mine. (I have always had a small personal practice in order to maintain my identity as a physician and healer.) As a member of the UCLA Faculty Medical Group, I accept referrals from the UCLA HIV/AIDS treatment unit, the apt acronym of which is "CARE" (Center for AIDS Research and Education). Thirty-three-year-old Paul Wagner was referred to me because of depression following the recent death of his partner, Jose, from AIDS. Paul himself was HIV seropositive with a low CD4 count. Just the year prior, he had joined the UCLA Department of Pediatrics faculty. Quiet and scholarly, he had been thrilled with his opportunity at UCLA. Not long after Jose's death, however, Paul fell ill and was soon unable to continue his biochemical research on congenital aminoacidurias.

Paul had grown up in New Jersey in a devoutly Roman Catholic home, with a mother of Irish descent and a father of German heritage. Jose's family, of Cuban origin, had fled Castro for Miami. In contrast to Paul, Jose was gregarious and extroverted. They made a perfect pair and were deeply in love. Paul and Jose had been together for 10 years, since ages 23 and 21, and had seen each other through their respective educations. They had traveled the world extensively. When Paul accepted the position at UCLA, Jose managed to find a good job at a brokerage firm in Los Angeles. As yet, however, they had relatively few friends in Southern California, having lived there only a year before Jose became ill. Jose's mother, trained as a nurse in Cuba, came to Los Angeles to take care of him and was joined by Paul's mother as his condition deteriorated rapidly. Jose's graveside service in Miami was attended only by his beloved mother, Paul, and Paul's parents, since Jose's Hispanically homophobic relatives refused to attend, hurting his mother deeply. Mrs. Wagner became Mrs. Dominguez's best friend.

From the outset, I really liked Paul—a bright, attractive, interesting, accomplished, open, sophisticated young man who was terribly sad. AIDS, that had developed only a month after Jose's death, was manifested by vision-threatening cytomegalovirus infection. Paul was being treated with foscarnet, a drug with miserable side effects, through a permanently implanted central venous line. Paul couldn't cry—even when he showed me a picture of Jose, who had possessed the type of striking Latin beauty most often found, I think, in Cubans. I placed Paul on antidepressant medication along with psychotherapy. Treatment worked. His mood lifted, and he decided that he wanted to go on with as full a life as possible. He even went out for dinner a couple of times with another man with AIDS, whom he had met in a support group. With my encouragement, Paul decided to visit old friends on the East Coast. There he became very ill with raging fevers. He returned and was hospitalized. Diagnosis was not clear but probably was MAI (a type of tuberculosis usually restricted to birds). Wasting syndrome and intractable diarrhea set in. Paul hated being in the hospital. His mother and, for a time, Jose's mother came to nurse him at home; his father commuted 6,000 miles every weekend from New Jersey. I made home visits and hospital visits during intermittent inpatient stays. (Paul's health insurance did not cover most of his psychiatric care, as is often the case. I surely didn't care.) His suffering was prolonged, and he became incontinent. His pretty, red-headed, freckled mother was at his bedside day and night.

Just before I left to lecture in Bogotá and Cali, Columbia, I told Paul that I would see him as soon as I returned in a week's time. He asked me to lean over the bed. He raised up and kissed me, saying, "I love you, Doc. Thanks." Transference (feelings from another source) displaced onto therapist? Overinvolvement by physician? If so, I don't give a damn. I did help. As I left the apartment for what I knew would be the last time, I said to Mr. and Mrs. Wagner, "I have seen so many wonderful, gifted young people tragically die from AIDS. Never have I seen such devoted and loving parents." I was sobbing as I walked to my car. Pam Wagner later wrote from New Jersey, "I don't know how to thank you for all you did for Paul and me. I know you will never forget him. Thank you for your flowers at church. They were beautiful. Paul is in Heaven and looking down on us. I miss him with all my heart." Pam was right; I'll never forget him. Perhaps you won't either.

I want to live long enough to discover some useful findings, biological as well as psychological, from my research on long-survival with HIV. I know its importance from the bedside and personally— in my heart, in my mind, in my blood.

DISTILLATIONS *

There are no simple answers in life. Psychoneuroimmunology certainly illustrates the complexity of the interrelationships between psychology and biology. In sum, what have I learned or distilled from what has been a complex, often difficult, generally interesting, and rather unusual life? Of course, since this book is a professional tale from a personal point of view, you have learned primarily about a portion of the professional side of my life. Admittedly, there is no clear line between what one has done and who one has been. My unconventional personal life no doubt relates to unorthodox approaches to professional challenges. I must agree with those who believe that wisdom accumulates with age. (Smart ass, rebellious youngsters do contribute to the evolution and dynamism of society, however.) Maybe it would do some good if I tried to state those adages in which I believe and those opinions that I hold, especially as evolved from experiences described in this saga. Since fallibility is intrinsic to man, each item must be taken with "a grain of salt". I make no apologies for my biases, which are honestly revealed. I'll start with two bits of advice that Paul Smith (journalist, mentor, and friend) gave me at age 19, the age at which I entered medical school and when this professional odyssey began.

---

* "Essences of anything": Webster's New Twentieth Century Dictionary of the English Language, Unabridged, Second Edition.

Never be in awe of anyone.

One is generally limited only by one's conception of oneself.

Physical and mental well-being are inextricably intertwined.

Humanization of medical care promotes healing.

Medicine needs new models of health and disease.

Psychiatry is in trouble because of lacking a framework to integrate neurobiology with psychodynamics; simple cause and effect thinking is not tenable.

Have a variety of strategies to cope with stress in order to lessen stressor-induced distress and, thus, to minimize distress-induced immunosuppression.

Being HIV seropositive or having AIDS or any other life-threatening illness should lead one to reassess one's life, find new meanings, and attend to one's needs—not to feel hopeless, pessimistic, or doomed.

Since expectations tend to be self-fulfilling, both in life and health, you may as well be optimistic.

Love is relevant to health.

Social attitudes, especially as they have an impact on self-esteem and self-expression, can affect health.

Don't let your doctor boss you around or permit him/her to ignore you.

If you get depressed for any period of time, get professional help.

Pay attention and give heed to inner messages from both your mind and your body.

Don't confuse assertiveness with hostility.

Stick up for yourself.

Be able to do favors; be able to ask for favors; be able to turn down unwanted favors.

Don't be freaked out if someone gets angry with you.

Express your feelings.

Tune in to what another person is experiencing.

There is no one type of good marriage or partnership.

Have at least one friend with whom you can be as honest as you are with yourself.

*Friendship, commitment, and love, not sex, make relation-
ships endure.*

The only thing you can count on in life is those who love you.

*The good teacher guides and enables rather than controls and
dominates.*

*Opposition to freedom of reproductive choice and simulta-
neously being tough on crime, which is often a result of
unwantedness and rejection, are logically incompatible.*

*Outcasts sometimes make greater contributions to social and
scientific progress than the well-accepted.*

Courage is more important than fame.

*Psychological strength arises from overcoming adversity, not
from having it easy; the strong person seeks challenges.*

*Even in a wartime situation, refuse to do what you find morally
repugnant or evil.*

*Assume that prejudice is based on ignorance before conclud-
ing that it is based on hate.*

*Freedom of speech is more important than "political correct-
ness".*

Interact with a variety of people whose ideas differ.

*If an idea of yours seems weird, don't give it up without first
trying to prove it, or else check with a psychiatrist.*

Recognize and seize opportunities.

Reasons are not excuses.

*Perseverance, patience, and tolerance of uncertainty and frus-
tration are critical to long-term success.*

Skepticism is not the same as negativism or cynicism.

*Beware of both authorities and iconoclasts; weigh the evidence
and think for yourself.*

*Don't mistake friendliness or flattery in the workplace for genu-
ine friendship or caring.*

Read a lot; make it varied.

*Be permissive toward your own feelings and fantasies; be re-
sponsible about your actual behaviors.*

Try to express appreciation and praise to colleagues, students, and loved ones.

Earlier stresses, like antigens, can be immunizing or sensitizing to new challenges.

Beware the person who is concerned about mankind but who doesn't give a damn about individual human beings.

Kindness and intelligence have no correlation.

Be wary of simple answers to complex questions.

Do not confuse role with identity.

Being child-like is not the same as being childish; preserve the former and eliminate the latter.

Try to find some humor in most situations.

Happiness cannot be sought directly; it is an automatic by-product of finding meaningfulness in life.

Try to develop the less well-developed aspects of your personality and abilities; don't always play to your strengths.

Violence is an epidemic that needs to be dealt with as a threat to public health.

Psychopaths make society sick; martyrs make themselves sick.

Some criminals are treatable.

The death penalty can be justified only by an argument of self-defense/prevention; it generally does not deter and may actually increase murder.

Sexuality and attraction are fluid.

It is important to be able to link love and sex; it is essential to be able to de-couple love from sex; it is optional to separate love and sex.

Gay men and lesbians should try to come out of the closet.

People (straight and gay) should accept the validity of bisexuality.

Like a tree, grow until you die.

Have a will to live, but don't fear death itself; it's inevitable— not necessarily when "predicted".

If possible, control you own dying process.

GLOSSARY OF SCIENTIFIC TERMS

ACTH—Adrenocorticotropic hormone, a peptide hormone released by the pituitary gland that stimulates the adrenal cortex to produce cortisol (corticosterone in rodents). It is also produced by lymphocytes and has immunoregulatory properties.

Activation markers—Cell surface molecular aggregates or soluble proteins that indicate that an immunologically competent cell is actively involved in an immunologic response.

Adjuvant—A substance that is capable of augmenting an immune response.

Adrenal gland—An endocrine gland located adjacent to the kidneys. Its outer cortex produces corticosteroids that contribute to metabolic activity and suppress immunity and inflammation. Its inner medulla produces epinephrine and norepinephrine as a result of the activity of the sympathetic nervous system; these substances act both as hormones and neurotransmitters.

Adrenocorticosteroid hormone—A nonprotein hormone in the chemical structure of the steroid produced by the outer portion of the adrenal gland, that has anti-inflammatory, glucose-mobilizing, and immunosuppressive properties.

Allergy (hypersensitivity)—An immune response to an otherwise nontoxic environmental substance that results in inflammatory secretory responses.

Antagonist—A drug or compound that is capable of preventing a response to a biologically active compound.

Antibody—The protein product of a B cell (plasma cell) which is capable of combining with the antigen that triggered its production. Antibodies are highly specific to a particular antigen.

Antigen—A substance that is recognized as being nonself and that is capable of eliciting an immune response. It is also capable of combining with antibodies and/or specific T cells.

Anxiety—Apprehension and nervousness resulting from an unconsciously perceived danger that is not proportional to a real current threat. Its biological concomitants are the same as those of fear.

Autoantibody—An antibody that attaches to self antigens and, thus, inappropriately fails to distinguish self from nonself.

Autoimmunity—An immune response directed against a person's own healthy cells, their constituents, or products.

Autonomic nervous system—The component of the nervous system that regulates a variety of internal organs and functions. It is comprised of the sympathetic and parasympathetic branches. The sympathetic branch tends to trigger emergency responses like rapid heart rate; the parasympathetic branch regulates normal biological activity like intestinal movement (peristalsis). Its central nervous system connections are in the hypothalamus.

B cells—Lymphocytes, and their precursors, that are antibody-producing. (Antibodies are actually secreted by plasma cells which differentiate from B cell progeny upon stimulation.)

Beta-endorphin—A type of neurotransmitter capable of producing biological and behavioral effects similar to those induced by morphine, an endogenous opioid.

Beta-2 microglobulin—A soluble activation marker that is a component of the major histocompatibility complex (MHC), proteins coded by genes that determine immunologic compatibility (self vs. nonself). The MHC is responsible, in part, for presentation of antigen to T cells for specific immunologic responses (Class 1 presents antigens to cytotoxic T cells; Class II is necessary for presentation to helper T cells).

Blastogenesis—Induction of the production of immature, reproducing lymphocytes (blast cells).

Catecholamines—Organic compounds that contain a benzene ring with two adjacent hydroxyl substituents (catechol). In studies of the nervous system, the term generally refers to dopamine, epinephrine, and norepinephrine.

Cellular immunity—A form of defense carried out by immunologic cells (macrophages, cytotoxic T cells, and natural killer cells) rather than by antibodies (humoral immunity).

Central nervous system (CNS)—The brain and spinal cord.

Character disorder—See Personality disorder.

Clone—Immunologically, a group of lymphocytes (B cell or T cell) with identical specificity that "expand" (reproduce) in response to an antigen corresponding to its specificity.

Complement—A group of proteins in serum that interact with combinations (complexes) of antigen-antibody and produce lysis (cell destruction) when the antigen is on an intact cell. Activation of the first complement protein leads to the sequential activation of other proteins in the group.

Concanavalin A (Con A)—A plant product (lectin) which is capable of stimulating predominantly T lymphocytes.

Conditioning (classical)—Learning that occurs when a stimulus that is naturally capable of producing a particular response is paired with a neutral stimulus. The neutral (conditioned) stimulus subsequently becomes capable of eliciting the same response as the naturally occurring one.

Coping—Engaging in adaptive behavior when facing a realistic challenge, often using a particular style (e.g., active, emotion-focused).

Cortex—The outer portion of an organ such as the adrenal gland or brain.

Corticosterone—The predominant glucocorticoid produced by the adrenal gland in rodents. At high concentrations it has been found to inhibit the immune system, although at low concentrations it is necessary in order for lymphocytes to function. It is released during the stress response and serves to mobilize glucose stores. It has anti-inflammatory properties.

Cytokines—Peptides that act as messengers between cells in paracrine (nearby but not adjacent like neurotransmitters) or endocrine (distant) manners. Lymphokines, which are produced by lymphocytes, are among the broader class of cytokines.

Cytoplasm—The part of a cell within the outer cell membrane that is not the nucleus.

Cytotoxic—Cells, cytokines, chemicals, or antibodies that are capable of causing damage to a target cell. Both T cells and natural killer cells can be cytotoxic.

Defenses (immunologic)—Mobilization of phagocytic, cytotoxic, and antibody-producing cells to kill invading microorganisms or neoplastic (cancer) cells.

Defenses (psychological)—Mental mechanisms used to help repress painful affects or conflicts.

Dementia—Reduction in intellectual faculties as a result of organic brain disease.

Depression (major depressive disorder)—A clinical syndrome consisting of lowered mood and self-esteem, retardation of psychological and motor activity, and alterations in sleep, appetite, and sex drive.

DNA—Desoxyribonucleic acid, the carrier of genetic information contained in genes, that is composed of a varied sequence of four molecules (nucleosides) comprising an "alphabet" plus the sugar desoxyribose. The nucleosides are arranged in two long strands as a cross-linked double helix within chromosomes in the nucleus of cells.

Dopamine—A neurotransmitter, dysfunctions of which have been linked to mental illness.

Dysphoria—Unpleasant emotions, "misery."

Ego—That portion of the psyche (mind) concerned with adaptation, coping, and defense.

Endocrine—Of, or relating to, the glandular secretion of chemical substances directly into the bloodstream to regulate cellular activity at distant sites.

Enzyme—A protein that acts as a biological catalyst, promoting a biochemical reaction without being destroyed.

Epinephrine—Hormone released by the central portion (medulla) of the adrenal gland which, along with norepinephrine, results from stimulating the sympathetic branch of the autonomic nervous system.

Fear—An appropriate emergency response proportional to an actual current danger. Its endocrine and autonomic consequences prepare for fight or flight.

Glucocorticoids—Steroids that are capable of mobilizing glucose and reducing inflammation. Cortisol is the primary form produced in humans. Corticosterone is the primary form produced in rodents.

Health maintenance organization (HMO)—Provides "managed care" on a capitation (per person enrolled) rather than a fee-for-service basis.

Helper T cells (CD4)—A type of T lymphocyte that facilitates antibody production by B cells (T helper-1) and killing by cytotoxic T cells (T helper-2). Both subtypes secrete specific cytokines.

Histocompatibility locus antigen (HLA)—The major determinant of an individual organism's immunologic "identity" that relates to compatibility for transplantation. Also called major histocompatibility complex (MHC).

Hormones—Chemical signals produced by endocrine glands to regulate distant cells.

Humoral immunity—Pertaining to soluble molecules (antibodies) that can attach to bacteria and viruses.

Hypothalamic-pituitary-adrenal axis (HPA)—The domino-like cascade whereby corticotropin-releasing hormone (CRH) from the hypothalamus of the brain stimulates the release of ACTH from the pituitary gland which in turn triggers glucocorticoid production by the adrenal gland. Glucocorticoids are steroids capable of mobilizing glucose and reducing inflammation. Cortisol is the primary form produced in humans while corticosterone is the primary form produced in rodents.

Hypothalamus—A structure located beneath the cerebral hemispheres of the brain which is responsible for regulating many endocrine functions, the autonomic nervous system, and immunity.

Immunoglobulin—Proteins containing two heavy and two light polypeptide chains, that are formed by plasma cells of the immune system. (Plasma cells differentiate from B cell progeny upon stimulation.) Antibodies are immunoglobulins.

> **IgA**—A type of immunoglobulin or antibody found in secretions.
>
> **IgD**—A type of immunoglobulin found in human B cells.
>
> **IgE**—The type of immunoglobulin that is primarily responsible for immediate hypersensitivity and allergic reactions in humans.
>
> **IgG**—The primary type of immunoglobulin or antibody present in humans.
>
> **IgM**—A relatively large immunoglobulin produced early during an immune response.

Immunosenescence—Deleterious effects upon the immune system associated with the aging process.

Innervation—The distribution of nerves to a particular tissue.

Interferon (INF)—Cytokines produced by a number of different cell types, especially the macrophage, that serve to help regulate the immune system and kill viruses. Interferon alpha is produced by lymphocytes (usually helper T cells). Interferon beta is produced by the macrophage and fibroblasts (cells that hold tissues together, giving them shape and providing structure for the specialized functioning cells of each organ).

Interleukins—Cytokines produced by any one of the different types of cells involved in an immune response, that serve functions of immunoregulation and may have central nervous system effects. (More are discovered continually; at least 15 have been identified as of this writing.) Some interleukins promote and others inhibit inflammation.

IL-1—An interleukin produced by macrophages that stimulates helper T cells to produce IL-2.

IL-2—An interleukin produced by helper T cells (specifically, T helper-1) that especially stimulates B cells and natural killer cells.

IL-4—An interleukin produced especially by T helper-2 cells that particularly stimulates cytotoxic T cells.

Large granular lymphocyte—Descriptive of the morphology of a lymphocyte that is usually a natural killer cell.

Ligand—A substance that binds to a receptor site and causes its activation.

Lymph node—A cluster of lymphocytes in a small organ along the lymphatic system where microorganisms can be trapped and immunologically destroyed.

Lymphocyte—A mononuclear white blood cell that responds in a relatively specific manner in response to antigens.

Lymphokines—Soluble products of lymphocytes that exert numerous biological functions during the course of an immune response. Such "messenger molecules" are more broadly termed cytokines.

Macrophage—A large phagocytic cell associated with fixed tissues in the body that also circulates in the form of a white blood cell, the monocyte. It is a key cell in the immune cascade, producing cytokines and presenting antigen to lymphocytes for the initiation of specific immune responses.

Metastasis—The migration (via the bloodstream or lymphatic system) and subsequent growth of malignant cells at sites distal to their origin.

Mitogen—A substance that is capable of inducing lymphocyte cell division.

Narcoanalytic—Under the influence of disinhibitory drug(s), usually sedative (such as amobarbital) and sometimes in combination with a stimulant (such as amphetamine).

Natural killer (NK) cells—A lymphocyte (that is not a B cell or a T cell) that can kill both virus-infected and cancer cells, only nonspecifically "knowing" self from nonself. It functions as a first line of defense and prevents metastasis.

Neopterin—A soluble activation marker produced by macrophages.

Neuroendocrine—The process whereby the brain regulates the biological activity of various endocrine glands throughout the body.

Neurohormone—A metabolic regulatory substance (hormone), the glandular secretion of which is controlled by the nervous system.

Neuroimmunomodulation—A synonym for psychoneuroimmunology that emphasizes its brain-->immune system limb and de-emphasizes its psychological component.

Neuroleptic—A drug with antipsychotic actions.

Neuron—A nerve cell capable of transmitting information.

Neuropeptide—A cytokine messenger molecule composed of amino acids that can be produced by neural cells. It can act locally or at a distance.

Neurosis—An older term for nonpsychotic symptomatic mental illnesses involving feelings or behaviors reflecting distortion but not lacking appreciation of reality. The feeling or behavior is not perceived by the individual as being part of his or her basic character.

Neurotransmitter—A chemical produced by neurons that transmits information between adjacent cells across a synapse, or gap junction.

Norepinephrine—A neurotransmitter and part of the sympathetic branch of the autonomic nervous system in the periphery.

Nucleus—The central portion of a cell containing genetic material (chromosomes, genes).

Opiate—A plant (poppy)-derived chemical that has analgesic (pain-reducing) and euphoria-inducing properties.

Opioid—A naturally occurring (endogenous) opiate peptide that has pain-relieving and often immunoregulatory properties.

Peptides—Sequences of amino acids that can serve as hormones as well as neurotransmitters.

Personality disorder—A condition involving psychopathological, or enduring, characteristics—in contrast to symptoms. These characteristics are considered by the individual to be part of, and not alien to, his or her basic nature.

Phagocytosis—The internalization of pathogens into leukocytes (white blood cells) and macrophages. This process usually results in the destruction of microorganisms.

Phytohemagglutinin (PHA)—A plant product (lectin) capable of stimulating predominantly T lymphocytes.

Pituitary gland—The master endocrine gland located in close proximity to the hypothalamus. Its hormones regulate a large number of endocrine glands throughout the body. It, in turn, is controlled by "release" hormones produced in the hypothalamus, which itself has close connections to the limbic system—a collection of brain regions that regulate emotion and memory (part of the "old" or "reptilian" brain).

Plasma—The liquid portion of blood that remains after removal of all cellular elements.

Plasma cells—B cells that are actively producing antibody.

Pokeweed mitogen (PWM)—A plant product capable of stimulating both B and T lymphocytes, predominantly the former.

Polyclonal expansion—Proliferation of lymphocytes responsive to a wide variety of antigens (nonspecifically).

Projective [test]—Utilizing an ambiguous stimulus, such as an inkblot (Rorschach) or picture (Thematic Apperception Test, or TAT), on which a person can "project" conscious or unconscious fantasies.

Proliferative response—A de-differentiation of lymphocytes to a less mature form (lymphoblast) that is followed by cell division and proliferation.

Protease—An enzyme that splits a protein or cleaves a fraction off a protein.

Psychoneuroimmunology—The study of the interrelationships among the brain, behavior, and immunity.

Psychosis—A major mental disorder involving either disorders of cognition, mood, or both, to the degree that there is significant loss of contact with reality.

Receptor—A peptide complex that is the attachment site for a communication molecule (e.g., neurotransmitter, hormone) or antigen that, after binding with its ligand, sets in motion intracellular metabolic events. A ligand is a substance that binds with a receptor.

Reverse transcriptase—The enzyme responsible for converting an RNA virus into DNA material so that the virus can be incorporated into the genome of a cell that then replicates the virus.

Rheumatoid factor—An autoantibody directed against IgG found in the sera of individuals who suffer from rheumatoid arthritis.

RNA—Ribonucleic acid, like DNA, a carrier of protein "manufacturing" information but containing the sugar ribose and generally residing in the cytoplasm of a cell.

Schizophrenia—A severe form of mental illness characterized by such features as abnormality in associations among thoughts, changes in affect, mixed emotions (ambivalence), withdrawal into fantasy life (autism), delusions, hallucinations, and lack of pleasure (anhedonia).

Serotonin—A type of neurotransmitter that has been implicated in regulating sensory perception and sleep, as well as body temperature.

Serum (pl. sera)—The liquid portion of blood that remains after clotting. (The clot contains blood cells and the protein elements that make up fibrin.)

State (psychological)—A transient psychological condition secondary to current situational factors.

Stress—An environmental or psychological challenge that disrupts homeostasis and requires adaptation, coping, and/or defense. It is perhaps better termed a "stressor", a challenge resulting in psychobiological "strain" or distress.

Suppressor T cell—A type of lymphocyte that reduces antibody production by B cells or activity of T cells.

Sympathetic nervous system—The division of the autonomic nervous system that is capable of mobilizing the body's energy resources. This usually occurs during periods of stress and arousal.

Synapse—A gap junction between neurons across which impulses are transmitted by chemical means.

T cell (T lymphocyte)—Lymphoid cells dependent upon the thymus gland for their maturation that participate in a large number of immune reactions. Among their many functions, immune T cells kill microorganisms as well as virus-infected and cancer cells and facilitate the activity of B cells and other T cells.

Thymus—A bi-lobed organ located beneath the sternum that regulates the development of T lymphocytes and "deletes" clones of lymphocytes that are self-directed (autoimmune).

Trait—An enduring psychological characteristic that can result from mastery of a developmental phase (e.g., trust) or an attempt to repair or deal with unresolved earlier issues (e.g., suspiciousness). *Styles* of coping with stress are traits.

Tumor necrosis factor (TNF)—A cytokine that is cytotoxic for tumor cells, has some antiviral and antiparasitic activity, has a variety of immunoregulatory properties, and can produce toxic shock syndrome. Its alpha form is produced by macrophages and its beta form by helper T cells.

Virulence—The degree of pathogenicity of a microorganism as indicated by death rate or severity of illness induced.

SELECTED READINGS

Scientific Books on Psychoneuroimmunology

Ader, R., Felten, D.L., Cohen, N. (eds.): *Psychoneuroimmunology, Third Edition.* Academic Press, San Diego, 2000.

Blalock, J.E. (ed.): *Neuroimmunoendocrinology, Second Edition.* Karger, Basel, 1992.

Buckingham, J.D., Gillies, G.E., Cowell, A.M. (eds.): *Stress, Stress Hormones and the Immune System.* John Wiley & Sons, London (UK), 1994

Frederickson, R.C.A., McGaugh, J.L., Felten, D.L. eds.): *Peripheral Signaling of the Brain. Role in Neural-Immune Interactions and Memory.* Hogrefe & Humber, Toronto, 1991.

Friedman, H., Klein, T., Friedman, A. (eds.): *Psychoneuroimmunology, Stress and Infection.* CRC Press, Boca Raton, FL, 1996.

Glaser, R. & Kiecolt-Glaser, J. (eds.): *Handbook of Human Stress and Immunity.* Academic Press, San Diego, CA, 1994.

Goodnick, P.J., Klimas, N.G. (eds.): *Chronic Fatigue and Related Immune Deficiency Syndromes.* American Psychiatric Press, Washington, DC, 1993.

Hall, N.R.S., Altman, F., Blumenthal, S.J. (eds.): *Mind-Body Interactions and Disease.* Health Dateline Press, Tampa, FL, 1995.

Hoffman-Goetz, L. (ed.): *Exercise and Immune Function.* CRC Press, Boca Raton, FL, 1996.

Husband , A.J. (ed.): *Psychoimmunology. CNS-Immune Interactions.* CRC Press, Boca Raton, FL, 1993.

Leonard, B.E. & Miller, K. (eds.): *Stress, The Immune System and Psychiatry.* John Wiley & Sons, Chichester, UK, 1995.

Lewis, C.E., O'Sullivan, C., Barraclough, G. (eds.): *The Psychoimmunology of Cancer.* Oxford University Press, New York, 1994.

Locke, S., Ader, R., Besedovsky, H., Hall, N., Solomon, G., Strom, T. (eds.): *Foundations of Psychoneuroimmunology.* Aldine, New York, 1985.

Pennebaker, J.W. (ed): *Emotion, Disclosure, & Health.* American Psycholological Association, Washington, D.C., 1995.

Powers, D.C., Morley, J.E., Coe, R.M. (eds.): *Aging, Immunity, and Infection.* Springer, New York, 1994.

Schmoll, H-J, Tewes, U., Plotnikoff, N.P. (eds.): *Psychoneuroimmunology.* Hogrefe & Huber, Lewiston, N.Y., 1991.

Solomon, G.F.: *Immune and Nervous System Interactions. An Annotated Bibliography Supporting Postulates on Communication Links, Similarities, and Implications.* Obtainable without fee from the website of the PsychoNeuroImmunology Research Society: pnirs.org.

Watson, R.R. (ed): *Alcohol, Drugs of Abuse, and Immune Functions.* CRC Press, Boca Raton, FL, 1996.

Friedman, H., Klein, T.W., Specter, S.C. (eds.): *Drugs of Abuse, Immunity, and Infection.* CRC Press, Boca Raton, FL, 1996.

Hoffman-Goetz, L. (ed.): *Exercise and Immune Function.* CRC Press, Boca Raton, FL, 1996.

Buckingham, J.C., Gillies, G.E., Cowell, A.-M. (eds.): *Stress, Stress Hormones and the Immune System.* John Wiley & Sons, Chichester (UK), 1997.

Henneberg, A.E., Kaschka, W. P., (eds.): *Immunological Alterations in Psychiatric Diseases.* Karger, Basel (Switzerland), 1997.

Watkins, A. (ed.): *Mind-Body Medicine. A Clinician's Guide to Psychoneuroimmunology.* Churchill Livingstone, New York, 1997.

Cardinali, E.P. & Fraschini, F. (eds): *Psycho-Immune Neuroendocrine Integrative Mechanisms.* Karger, Basel, 1998.

Oomura, Y. & Hori, T. (eds): *Brain and Biodefense.* Karger, Basel, 1998.

Rabin, B.S.: *Stress, Immune Function, and Health. The Connection.* Wiley-Liss, New York, 1999.

Schedlowski, M. & Tewes, U. (eds): *Psychoneuroimmunology. An Interdisciplinary Introduction.* Klewer Academic. Plenum, London, 1999

Goodkin   K.   and   Visser,   A.P.   (eds.): *PSYCHONEUROIMMUNOLOGY. Stress, Mental Disorders, and Health.* American Psychiatric Press, Washington, D.C., 2000.

Nott, K.H., Vedhara, K. (eds.): *Psychosocial and Biomedical Interactions in HIV Infection.* Harwood Academic Publishers, Amsterdam, the Netherlands, 2000.

Harbuz, M. (ed.): *Stress and Immunity: The Neuroendocrine Link>* Balliere's London, 2000.

Books Relevant to Psychiatry, Psychotherapy, Mind/Body, Vietnam, Criminology, & Sexuality (books from which cases or material were drawn are marked with an asterisk)

Antonovsky, A.: *Unraveling the Mystery of Health.* Jossey-Bass, San Francisco, 1988.

Brende, J.L. & Parson, E.R.: *Vietnam Veterans.* Plenum, New York, 1985.

Bugliosi, V. with Gentry, C.: *Helter Skelter.* W.W. Norton, New York, 1974. *(Manson)*

*Callan, M.: *Surviving AIDS.* Harper Collins, New York, 1990.

Cousins, N.: *Anatomy of an Illness.* W.W. Norton, New York, 1979.

*Cousins, N.: *Head First: The Biology of Hope.* E.P. Dutton, New York, 1988.

*Daniels, D.N., Gilula, M.F., Ochberg, F. (eds.): *Violence and the Struggle for Existence.* Little Brown, Boston, 1970.

*Denerell, W.: *Fatal Cruise.* McClelland & Stewart, Toronto, 1991. *(Murder at sea case)*

Figley, C.R. (ed.): *Stress Disorders among Vietnam Veterans.* Brunner/ Mazel, New York, 1978.

Fletcher, B.C.: *Work, Stress, Disease, and Life Expectancy.* John Wiley & Sons, Chichester, UK, 1991.

Fromm, E.: *The Anatomy of Human Destructiveness.* Holt, Rinehart & Winston, New York, 1973.

Goldberg, J.Ge.: *Psychotherapeutic Treatment of Cancer Patients.* Free Press, New York, 1981.

Hahn, R.A.: *Sickness and Healing.* Yale University Press, New Haven, CT, 1995. *(Anthropology)*

Hendin, H. & Haas, A.P.: *Wounds of War.* Basic Books, New York, 1984.

Hirshberg, C & Barasch, M.I.: *Remarkable Recovery.* Riverhead Books, New York, 1995.

*Horowitz, M.J.: *Stress Response Syndromes. Second Edition.* Jason Aronson, Northvale, NJ, 1986.

*Isaac, R.J. & Armat, V.C.: *Madness in the Streets.* Free Press, New York, 1990. *(Homeless mentally ill)*

Johnson, R. & Toch, H. (eds.): *The Pains of Imprisonment.* Sage, Beverly Hills, CA, 1982.

*Kangas, J.A. & Solomon, G.F.: *The Psychology of Strength.* Prentice-Hall, Englewood Cliffs, NJ, 1975.

Karon, B.P. & Vanderbos, G.R.: *Psychotherapy of Schizophrenia.* Jason Aronson, New York, 1995.

Kepner, J.I.: *Body Process.* Jossey-Bass, San Francisco, 1987. *(Integrating psychotherapy and bodywork)*

Klein, F. & Wolf, T.J. (eds.): *Bisexuality: Theory and Research.* Hayworth Press, New York, 1985.

Lappé M.: *The Tao of Immunology.* Plenum Trade, New York, 1997.

Lazarus, R.S. & Folkman, S.: *Stress, Appraisal, and Coping.* Springer, New York, 1984.

Lifton, R.J.: *Home From the War*. Simon and Schuster, New York, 1973.

*Livsey, C.: *The Manson Women*. Richard Marek, New York, 1980. *(Leslie Van Houten case)*

*Lunde, D.T.: *Murder and Madness*. W.W. Norton, New York, 1975. *(Kemper case)*

Malcolm, J.: *Psychoanalysis: The Impossible Profession*. Alfred A. Knopf, New York, 1981.

Meloy, J.R.: *The Psychopathic Mind*. Jason Aronson, Northvale, N.J., 1988.

Menninger, K.: *The Crime of Punishment*. Viking Press, New York, 1966.

Meshad, S.: *Captain for Dark Mornings*. Creative Image Associates, Playa del Rey, CA, 1982. *(Vietnam)*

Mitford, J.: *Kind and Usual Punishment*. Alfred A. Knopf, New York, 1973. (Prisons)

Murphy, M.: *The Future of the Body*. Jeremy P. Tarcher, Los Angeles, 1992. *(Human potentiality)*

Ornstein, R. & Swencionis (eds.): *The Healing Brain*. Guilford Press, New York, 1990.

Radelet, M.L. (ed.): *Facing the Death Penalty*. Temple University Press, Philadelphia, 1989.

Reid, W.H. (ed.): *The Treatment of Antisocial Syndromes*. Van Nostrand Reinhold, New York, 1981.

Rogers, K.P.: *For One Sweet Grape*. Playboy Press, Chicago, 1974. *(Criminal autobiography)*

Shields, R.W.: *A Cure of Delinquents*. International Universities Press, London, 1962; New York, 1971.

Singer, M.T. with Lalich, J.: *Cults in our Midst*. Jossey-Bass, San Francisco, 1995.

Smith, A.B. & Berlin, L.: *Treating the Criminal Offender. Second Edition*. Prentice-Hall, Englewood Cliffs, NJ, 1987.

*Solomon, J.C.: *A Synthesis of Human Behavior*. Grune & Stratton, New York, 1954.

*Stürup, G.K.: *Treating the "Untreatable"*. Johns Hopkins Press, Baltimore, 1968. (Offender treatment)

*Temoshok, L. & Baum, A. (eds.): *Psychosocial Perspectives on AIDS*. Lawrence Erlbaum, Hillsdale, NJ, 1990.

Temoshok, L. & Dreher, H.: *The Type C Connection*. Random House, New York, 1992.

*Temoshok, L., Van Dyke, C., Zegans, L. (eds.): *Emotions in Health and Illness*. Grune & Stratton, New York, 1983.

Vaillant, G.: *The Wisdom of the Ego*. Harvard University Press, Cambridge, MA, 1993.

*Wallerstein, R.S.: *The Doctorate in Mental Health*. University Press of America, Lanham, MD, 1991.

Weatherall, D.: *Science and the Quiet Art*. W.W. Norton, New York, 1995. *(Academia)*

Weinberg, M.S., Williams, C.J., Pryor, D.W.: *Dual Attraction*. Oxford University Press, Oxford, 1994. (Bisexuality)

Weiner, H.: *Perturbing the Organism*. University of Chicago Press, Chicago, 1992.

Winiarski, M.G.: *AIDS-related Psychotherapy*. Pergamon Press, New York, 1991. (Psychology)

Yalom, I.D.: *Love's Executioner and Other Tales of Psychotherapy*. Basic Books, New York, 1989.

Moyers, B.: *Healing and the Mind*. Doubleday, New York, 1993.

O'Regan, B, Hirshberg, C., Lewis, M., McNeil, B., Franklin, M: *The Heart of Healing*. Turner Publishing, Atlanta, 1993.

Martin, P.: *The Healing Mind. The Vital Links between Brain and Behavior, Immunity and Disease*. St. Martin's Press, New York, 1997.

Firestein, B. (ed.): *Bisexuality. The Pyschology and Politics of an Invisible Minority*. Sage Publications, Thousand Oaks, CA, 1996.

Sternberg, E.M.: *The Balance Within. The Science Connecting Health and Emotions*. W. H. Freeman and Company, New York, 2000.